Dr Michelle Harvie and Professor Tony Howell work at the Genesis Breast Cancer Prevention Centre, part of The University Hospital of South Manchester NHS Foundation Trust. Genesis Breast Cancer Prevention is the only breast cancer charity in the UK entirely dedicated to prevention. Because weight is a significant factor in the risk of developing breast cancer, Dr Harvie and Prof Howell have spent years researching and developing the optimum diet to help people lose weight quickly and easily and to keep off weight lost in the longer term. This incredibly effective diet is the result of their clinical research.

Dr Michelle Harvie is an award-winning research dietitian. For the last 18 years she has specialised in optimum diet and exercise strategies for weight loss and preventing breast cancer and its recurrence. Her findings have been published in many major scientific journals. She was awarded the British Dietetic Association Rose Simmonds Award for best published dietetic research in 2005, Manchester City Council's 2007 International Women's Day Award for Women in Science, and the National Association for the Study of Obesity Best Practice Award for best published obesity research in 2010.

Prof Tony Howell is Professor of Medical Oncology at the University of Manchester. He has specialised in treating breast cancer for over 30 years and now focuses on pharmacological and lifestyle measures to prevent breast cancer. He is Research Director of Genesis Breast Cancer Prevention and has published over 600 scientific papers and book chapters, mainly concerning the biology of the breast and the treatment and prevention of breast cancer.

All author proceeds from the sale of this book will go to Genesis Brea **K charity entirely** **dedica** **registered** **charit**

D0610774

Praise for The 2-Day Diet

'Clinically proven and guarantees weight loss'
Daily Mail

'Revolutionary and clinically proven'
Good Housekeeping

'Easy to follow and stick to'
Jenni Murray

'The key to easier – and longer lasting – weight loss'
Red

'Surprisingly effective results'
Bella

the

2
day diet

The
QUICK & EASY edition

Dr Michelle Harvie & Prof Tony Howell

Vermilion
LONDON

3 5 7 9 10 8 6 4 2

First published in 2014 by Vermilion, an imprint of Ebury Publishing
A Random House Group company

The Random House Group Limited Reg. No. 954009
Addresses for companies within the Random House Group can be found at
www.randomhouse.co.uk

The Random House Group Limited supports the Forest Stewardship Council® (FSC®),
the leading international forest-certification organisation. Our books carrying the
FSC label are printed on FSC®-certified paper. FSC is the only forest-certification
scheme supported by the leading environmental organisations, including Greenpeace.
Our paper procurement policy can be found at www.randomhouse.co.uk/environment

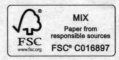

Designed and set by seagulls.net
Printed in the UK by CPI Group (UK) Ltd, Croydon, CR0 4YY

ISBN 9780091954857
To buy books by your favourite authors and register for offers visit www.randomhouse.co.uk

Contents

Contents

Introducing
The 2-Day Diet

If you are someone who has tried, and failed, to lose weight, or you've shed the extra pounds, only to pile them back on again – this is the book for you. The 2-Day Diet is a brand new, research-based approach to weight loss, which can work for you whether you've been struggling with your weight for years or have only just made the decision to lose weight. The 2-Day Diet is simple: you diet for just two consecutive days a week and eat normally for the other five. You don't have to fast, skip meals or feel hungry. It is a flexible, easy to follow approach that will help you to shift your unwanted pounds even when other diets have failed. Designed by research dietitian Dr Michelle Harvie and research director Prof Tony Howell at Genesis Breast Cancer Prevention, The 2-Day Diet has been rigorously tested in clinical trials, is proven to work and is nutritionally balanced to meet all your body's needs.

Why weight matters

Being overweight is bad for us. It increases the risk of heart disease, stroke, type 2 diabetes, dementia, 12 different cancers and makes you more prone to arthritis, indigestion, gallstones, stress, anxiety, depression, infertility and sleep problems. In fact being very overweight (3 stone/19 kg above your healthy weight) is as harmful as smoking and can reduce your life expectancy by eight years. Just as important, being overweight limits your years of good health. In the UK women live to the age of 82, on average, but their good health only lasts until their mid sixties. Similarly men live to 78, on average, with good health until the age of 64.[1]

This new, scientifically tested approach to weight loss, backed by eight years of research, will help you to:

▶ Escape day-in day-out calorie counting and still lose weight

▶ Cut down for two days a week

▶ Eat normally for the other five days

▶ Lose weight faster and more effectively than on a conventional seven-day, low-calorie diet

▶ Target loss of fat and not muscle

▶ Retrain your appetite so you can move away from over-eating and unhealthy food cravings

▶ Achieve successful weight loss even when everything else has failed

▶ Keep the weight off long term

▶ Achieve major health benefits including a reduction in your risk of type 2 diabetes, heart disease and some cancers

Do you need to lose weight?

If your favourite jeans feel a bit tight, or you've moved up a size or two, the answer might be obvious. But how can you tell whether your weight could be harming your health? Health problems arise from carrying too much fat – especially fat stored in the wrong places (in the abdomen or muscles). So just looking in the mirror or standing on the scales may not immediately tell you the answer. The steps below should help give you a better picture of your health.

Step 1: Work out your Body Mass Index (BMI)

BMI is the most common way of calculating whether or not you are a healthy weight. BMI is calculated as:

Your weight (in kg) ÷ your height (in metres squared)

If your BMI is 18.5 to 24.9 your weight is normal. A BMI of 25–29.9 is overweight with increased health risks and a BMI of 30 or more is classified as 'obese', with even greater health risks. The healthiest BMI is around 20–22.

So, for example, the average woman in the UK weighs (71.2 kg) (11 stone 3 lb) and is 1.62 m (5 ft 4 in) tall, which means she has a BMI of 27.1 (and is therefore overweight!)

You can find an online BMI calculator at www.thetwoday diet.co.uk.

Step 2: Calculate your percentage of body fat

Two people of the same height, weight and BMI may have vastly different amounts of body fat and, as a result, very different health risks. An inactive woman with a BMI of 27 might have as much as 45 per cent of her weight as fat, while another with the same BMI might be an athlete with lots of muscle and only 19 per cent of her weight as fat. As a general rule, women should have 20–34 per cent of their body weight as fat and men should have 8–25 per cent. You will find a Body Fat Ready Reckoner, which estimates your body fat from your weight, height, age and sex at www.thetwodaydiet.co.uk. You can also buy stand-on scales that measure body fat using a tiny electric current, for around £30–£50. Stand-on scales send a current through your lower body, and are more accurate than hand-held body fat monitors that just measure your arms, although they are still not foolproof.

Step 3: Check your waistline

Some people gain weight on their bottoms and thighs ('pears'), while others pile it on around their waist ('apples'). If you're an 'apple', with fat around your middle, you probably also have extra fat stored on the inside, around the vital organs inside your abdomen. This internal fat is very dangerous for your health, causing inflammation in the body, which in turn increases the risk of type 2 diabetes, heart disease, stroke and possibly some cancers.

'I was lethargic, always hungry and unfit. With a family history of diabetes and high blood pressure, I needed to do something before it was too late. The diet helped me lose three stone, I am so much fitter and my energy levels have soared.' Greg, 49

Warning

You should not attempt The 2-Day Diet if you are a child, a teenager, pregnant, breastfeeding or have an eating disorder. The moderately high levels of protein in this diet may pose problems for anyone with kidney disease or anyone at risk of kidney disease. If you have diabetes, any other medical condition or if you are taking medication, seek advice from your GP before embarking on any diet and exercise programme.

About the diet

The 2-Day Diet is based on eight years of research, working with overweight women who were desperate to lose weight to reduce their risk of breast cancer. Being overweight significantly increases breast cancer risk while our research, and that of others, shows that losing as little as 4.5 kg (10 lb) can cut the risk by 25 to 40 per cent.[2] But as anyone who has dieted knows, losing weight – and keeping it off – can be difficult. Most people stick with a diet for three to six months and lose around 6.4 kg (1 stone) but eight out of ten dieters put most of the weight back on again.[3] This process of losing and regaining the weight can become pretty demoralising so we set out to develop a diet that would help people to do it differently.

'I am losing around 2 lb a week with The 2-Day Diet so it's easy to keep motivated and I feel great knowing this diet also has so many health benefits. It fits really well into family life – my husband and kids enjoy the recipes too.'
Helen, 37

As intriguing animal studies emerged about the potential health benefits of restricting calories for a few days of the week[4,5] we decided to develop a diet which involved dieting for just two days of the week and tested it on groups of dieters. This was a pioneering approach as nobody had ever tried this pattern of eating to help people lose weight.

We decided on a 2-Day Diet as we thought it would be do-able, but last for long enough to reduce the overall calorie intake necessary for people to lose weight. At the same time it would enable them to retrain their appetite and diet habits and provide a long enough period of a lower calorie intake to achieve a better balance of hormones and healthier cells in the body.

We looked at how 2–Day Dieters fared compared to dieters who did a standard reduced-calorie diet every day of the week. The results showed us that when it comes to weight loss, 2-Day Dieting works better and often succeeds where other diets fail. It seems to be more manageable and delivers better health benefits.

What's more, when we followed people over the longer term, 2-Day Dieters had kept their weight off and changed their eating habits. In one study, we followed 2-Day Dieters for 12–15 months after they first started the diet. We found that they hadn't regained weight and had maintained their healthier lower levels of cholesterol and insulin by following the diet for just one day a week. Insulin plays a vital role in regulating sugar levels in the body and poor insulin function is at the root of many diseases such as type 2 diabetes, heart disease, some cancers and possibly dementia. In our studies, the 2-Day Dieters had much greater reductions in insulin than seven-day dieters throughout the week and particularly after their two low-carb, low-calorie diet days, when their insulin levels dropped even further.[6]

You can expect to see rapid results on The 2-Day Diet and lose up to 2 kg (4 lb) of fat per week. The diet is designed to help the body to quickly shift to *burning* fat rather than storing it. In our clinical trials 2-Day Dieters lost fat about one and a half times more quickly than those on a conventional seven-day, calorie-controlled diet, and lost more centimetres around their waists, which is where the fat most harmful to your health is stored.

We've included plenty of protein on The 2-Day Diet for several reasons. Firstly, research suggests that our appetites are fundamentally controlled by our need for protein. The body will keep telling you that you are hungry until you have eaten enough of it. Because you'll be enjoying filling proteins and healthy fats on your diet days, you'll be losing weight without ever feeling hungry.

Protein is also what helps to maintain muscle mass when you diet (which can be lost if you don't get the balance right when dieting).

Dieters who have successfully lost weight seem to be more likely to overeat and regain weight if they lost a lot of muscle as well as fat when they lost weight.

Protein foods are also helpful to dieters because they burn an extra 65–70 calories to absorb and digest them.

There are plenty of protein options for vegetarians on The 2-Day Diet; just refer to the vegetarian section on page 145.

So now you know the background, let's get started!

'The 2-Day Diet was a simple, well laid-out plan that changed my approach to what I eat and when. It is a new way of life and it's easy.' George, 46

What is The 2-Day Diet?

▶ Two consecutive diet days and five days of normal eating.

▶ Low enough in calories to enable you to lose weight, but without leaving you feeling hungry.

▶ Nutritionally balanced so that all your protein, vitamin and mineral requirements are met.

▶ Easy to fit into a normal, busy lifestyle and family life.

▶ A diet that works equally well for men and women and is suitable for vegetarians.

How do I do the two diet days?

▶ You eat a low-carb diet with 650–1000 calories per diet day.

▶ You are allowed plenty of high-protein foods, healthy fats, low-fat dairy foods, vegetables and some fruit.

▶ You avoid high-carbohydrate foods.

▶ Try to do your two diet days back-to-back to get the full benefits of the diet. Our research found that doing the two days together makes dieting easier and ensures that you get around to doing the second day. Doing two days together also means your body has a longer spell with lower levels of hormones, which may provide extra health benefits.

▶ Stay well-hydrated and drink at least 2 litres (4 pints) of fluid a day.

▶ There is no need to take a vitamin supplement.

▶ Eat the recommended portions of protein, fats, low-fat dairy, vegetables and fruit. The tables in the back of this book include lots of examples of different foods and an at-a-glance guide to how to work out your portions.

How much can I eat on my two diet days?

The 2-Day Diet allows you a specific number of portions of protein, fat, low-fat dairy foods, fruit and vegetables on your diet days as set out below.

Portions on your two diet days

Men	Portions
Carbohydrate	0
Protein	Minimum 4, maximum 14
Fats	Maximum 6
Low-fat Dairy	3 (recommended)
Vegetables	5 (recommended)
Fruit	1 (recommended)

Women	Portions
Carbohydrate	0
Protein	Minimum 4, maximum 12
Fats	Maximum 5
Low-fat Dairy	3 (recommended)
Vegetables	5 (recommended)
Fruit	1 (recommended)

People can feel confused by the portions and assume that a 2-Day Diet 'portion' is the same as the amount of that food you would eat for a meal. In fact the portion sizes in this book are generally much smaller than a typical meal-size serving. A 2-Day Diet chicken portion, for example, is 30 g (1 oz). A typical chicken breast weighs 120–180 g (4–6 oz) so contains between four and six portions.

These smaller portion sizes mean that you can tailor the diet to the amount you need to eat and your appetite and ensure that your diet contains the right balance of nutrients.

Protein foods are an essential part of the diet and you need to have a minimum amount of protein on your diet days, but because it is equally important that you don't overeat we have set a maximum limit. Whether you have the minimum or the maximum, or find that the right amount for you is somewhere in between is up to you.

The two diet days also allow a certain amount of healthy fats. These aren't essential on the diet days so if you want to reduce them to a minimum or cut them out altogether that is fine. However, you should include healthy fats on the five non-diet days.

Most dieters quickly discover how many protein and fat portions they need to avoid feeling hungry, and how best to spread them out through the day, and tend to keep to this. You may feel hungrier on some days than others so adapt your portions accordingly. The most important thing to remember on your two diet days is to have the minimum recommended portions for protein, dairy, fruit and vegetables.

You will find two weeks of meal plans covering your two diet and five non-diet days for both meat eaters and vegetarians on page 156. We have found that dieters find the meal planners very helpful, particularly in the early days of the diet. The planners are based on an average number of 2-Day Diet portions of protein and fat, low-fat dairy, fruit and vegetables and will help you to get to grips with the diet.

Once you feel confident about how The 2-Day Diet works, start experimenting with some different recipes – you will find plenty of delicious suggestions on pages 73–134 – or play around with the number of portions you have at each meal to find what works best for you (see The 2-Day Diet portion guides in Appendix A).

What can I eat on my diet days?

Healthy protein foods (e.g. chicken, fish, seafood, eggs, lean meat, tofu, Quorn, textured vegetable protein (TVP), tempeh or soya beans). Portion sizes are 30–60 g (1–2 oz) depending on the food. (See Appendix A for detailed portion information.)

▶ Women are allowed a minimum of 4 and maximum of 12 protein portions per day.

▶ Men are allowed a minimum of 4 and maximum of 14 protein portions per day.

Healthy fats (e.g. rapeseed oil, olive oil, nuts or avocado). A portion is a dessertspoon of oil or nuts, or ¼ avocado.

▶ Women are allowed a maximum of 5 portions per day.

▶ Men are allowed a maximum of 6 portions per day.

Low-fat dairy foods (e.g. cheese, milk, yoghurt). A portion is 195 ml (⅓ pint) of semi-skimmed or skimmed milk, 150 g (5 oz) yoghurt or 30 g (1 oz) low-fat cheese.

▶ Women and men should have 3 portions per day.

Fruit (low-carb, e.g. melon, berries, apricots).

▶ Women and men should have 1 piece of low-carb fruit per day.

Vegetables (low-carb, e.g. broccoli, tomatoes, mushrooms)

▶ Women and men should have 5 portions or bowlfuls of low-carb vegetables or salad per day.

Drinks

▶ Women and men should have at least 2 litres (4 pints) of water, tea, coffee, or other sugar-free or low-calorie drinks per day.

Snack ideas for your diet days

▶ Olives
▶ Handful of nuts (not chestnuts) or roast soya beans
▶ Fruit from the allowed list
▶ Vegetable crudités, such as celery, cucumber, green peppers, mangetout, spring onion and cherry tomatoes, with salsa, low-fat hummus or guacamole

▶ Plain or diet yoghurt

▶ Bowl of soup i.e. cauliflower, Chinese vegetable soup with tofu, see pages 77–79

▶ Salad or cooked vegetables with 75 g (2½ oz) of cottage cheese, 1 tablespoon of low-fat cream cheese or 1 tablespoon of low-fat hummus

▶ Half a 200 g (7 oz) pot of cottage cheese

▶ Smoothie made with skimmed or semi-skimmed milk, yoghurt and one piece of fruit

▶ Half a 120 g (4 oz) tin of sardines or pilchards

▶ Salty drink (see page 15)

▶ Sautéed tofu or chicken strips lightly fried in spices

▶ Boiled egg

▶ Avocado, mozzarella, tomato and basil skewers or stacks

▶ Celery sticks filled with low-fat cream cheese

▶ Asparagus spears dipped in soft-boiled egg

▶ Sugar-free jelly

▶ Ice lolly made from frozen, diluted, sugar-free squash

Flavourings

You can use the following flavourings freely on diet days:

▶ Lemon juice

▶ Fresh or dried herbs

▶ Spices or black pepper

▶ Mustard

▶ Horseradish

▶ Vinegars

▶ Garlic, fresh or pre-chopped

▶ Chilli, fresh or dried

▶ Soy sauce

▶ Miso paste

▶ Fish sauce

▶ Worcester sauce

Below are typical diet days based on an average amount of protein and fat. If women are still hungry, they can add up to three more portions of protein (for example, a bigger piece of chicken in the stir-fry or an extra rasher or two of bacon at breakfast) and another fat portion (for example, half an avocado with your lunchtime salad).

Men can add up to three more portions of protein (for example, more smoked salmon in the salad, an extra rasher of bacon with your breakfast and a tablespoon of hummus as a snack). You can also have one more extra fat portion, so you might want to have an extra handful of nuts.

If you find that you're too full, replace the mid-afternoon nuts with vegetable crudités and use just one egg for breakfast. Remember though: don't go below four protein portions. If you want to cut fats out on your diet days you can skip the nuts, oil and avocado. You can find a full guide to 2-Day Diet portion sizes in Appendix A.

All about salt

On your diet days you will be fat-burning and passing water and electrolytes so you must drink plenty (2 litres/4 pints). You should also include some salt, but you don't need huge amounts. There is some naturally occurring salt in dairy foods, fish and seafood.

If you develop headaches on diet days, you may need a little more water and salt. Try including a salty food, such as smoked fish, bacon, ham, olives, feta cheese, salted nuts or include one of the following:

- ½ stock cube or 2 teaspoons bouillon as a drink or in cooking

- 1 tablespoon soy sauce

- 1 teaspoon yeast extract or meat stock with hot water

- 3 teaspoons gravy powder or granules dissolved in hot water

Do not include a salty drink or salty foods if you are taking a water tablet for high blood pressure. Too much salt is bad for blood pressure and bones so limit these salty foods on the non-diet days to just one serving per week.

Typical Diet Day For Women

	2-Day Diet Portions				
Breakfast	Protein	Fat	Dairy	Fruit	Veg
Half a grapefruit				1	
Scrambled eggs made with 2 eggs	2				
1 grilled tomato					1
Mid-morning					
A matchbox-sized piece of Edam (30 g/1 oz)			1		
Lunch					
90 g (3 oz) smoked salmon	3				
¼ avocado		1			
Bowl of salad leaves (80 g/3 oz)					1
Dressing made from 1 tsp olive oil and a squeeze of lemon juice		½			
Mid-afternoon					
Handful of cashews (15 g/½ oz)		2			
Evening meal					
Chicken stir-fry made with 120 g (4 oz) chicken breast	4				
1 tsp rapeseed oil Handful of mangetout (80 g/3 oz) 6 baby sweetcorn (80 g/3 oz) 2 florets broccoli (80 g/3 oz)		½			3
Supper					
3 tbsp low-fat Greek or diet yoghurt			1		
200 ml (7 fl oz) of milk in tea and coffee during the day			1		
TOTAL IN DAY	9	4	3	1	5

Typical Diet Day For Men

Breakfast	2-Day Diet Portions				
	Protein	Fat	Dairy	Fruit	Veg
Half a grapefruit				1	
Scrambled eggs made with 2 eggs	2				
1 grilled tomato					1
1 rasher lean grilled bacon	1				
Mid-morning					
A matchbox-sized piece of Edam (30 g/1 oz)			1		
Lunch					
90 g (3 oz) smoked salmon	3				
½ avocado		2			
Bowl of salad leaves (80 g/3 oz)					1
Dressing made from 1 tsp olive oil and a squeeze of lemon juice		½			
Mid-afternoon					
Handful of cashews (15 g/½ oz)		2			
Evening meal					
Chicken stir-fry made with 150 g (5 oz) chicken breast	5				
1 tsp rapeseed oil Handful of mangetout (80 g/3 oz) 6 baby sweetcorn (80 g/3 oz) 2 florets broccoli (80 g/3 oz)		½			3
Supper					
3 tbsp low-fat Greek or diet yoghurt			1		
200 ml (7 fl oz) milk in tea and coffee during the day			1		
TOTAL IN DAY	11	5	3	1	5

Here is a blank version of the 2-Day Diet Tracker for you to use yourself. You can also find the table on The 2-Day Diet website (www.thetwodaydiet.co.uk) to download and print.

	2-Day Diet Portions				
Breakfast	Protein	Fat	Dairy	Fruit	Veg
Mid-morning					
Lunch					
Mid-afternoon					
Evening meal					
Supper					
TOTAL IN DAY					

Stick to the plan

Don't be tempted to devise your own two-day low-calorie diet. It will be harder to do because it will almost certainly leave you feeling hungry and a 'made-up' diet that isn't nutritionally balanced is unlikely to deliver the same health or weight-loss benefits as The 2-Day Diet.

How do I do five non-diet days?

▶ For the non-diet days of The 2-Day Diet we recommend a healthy Mediterranean diet, which includes wholegrain carbohydrate foods, lots of vegetables, fish, poultry, beans, pulses, fruit, nuts, healthy fats and oils, low-fat dairy foods and small amounts of lean, red meat. (See the Ready Reckoners on page 164 and the food lists on page 137.)

▶ Eat plenty of healthy protein foods on these non-diet days to help to fill you up, stop you overeating and maximise your weight loss.

▶ Have plenty of high-fibre carbs on non-diet days, including cereals, rye crispbreads, wholemeal pasta, pulses, vegetables and fruit. These help to keep you full, keep your bowel healthy and keep your blood sugar stable, which reduces the chances of overeating.

▶ The Mediterranean diet is packed with disease-fighting antioxidants, vitamins and flavonoids as well as fibre and has been shown to lower the risk of heart disease and type 2 diabetes. It may even protect against some cancers and Alzheimer's disease.[7]

▶ Don't be tempted to overeat, eat junk food or high-sugar food or drinks on non-diet days. Follow the guidelines to give yourself the best possible chance of successful weight loss.

▶ You can have treats such as alcohol and chocolate, but limit them to two or three times a week on non-diet days.

How much can I eat on my non-diet days?

It goes without saying that the diet won't work if you overeat on your non-diet days. One of the most exciting and consistent findings with The 2-Day Diet is that most people don't overeat and naturally restrict themselves on their non-diet days. Just to ensure that you don't eat too much, we've provided Ready Reckoners to show how much you should eat (see Appendix D, page 164). These give maximum amounts for men and women according to age and weight. On non-diet days we recommend you include protein, dairy, fruit, vegetables and include some healthy fats. Below you'll find examples of a typical non-diet day for men and women.

Typical Non-Diet Day for Women

	2-Day Diet Portions					
Breakfast	**Carbs**	**Protein**	**Fat**	**Dairy**	**Fruit**	**Veg**
Bowl of porridge made with 2 heaped tbsp porridge oats (40 g/1½ oz) and 200 ml (7 fl oz) semi-skimmed milk Cup of tea	2			1		
Mid-morning						
Banana					1	
Cup of coffee						
Lunch						
Tuna pasta salad						
60 g (2 oz) wholemeal pasta twists (dry weight)	2					
180 g (6 oz) tuna (drained weight) in spring water		4				
Bowl of lettuce, 10 cherry tomatoes, ¼ pepper						3
1 tbsp low-fat mayonnaise			1			
Fruit yoghurt 150 g (5 oz)				1		
Low-calorie drink						
Mid-afternoon						
Handful of pistachio nuts 15 g (½ oz)		2				
Cup of tea						
Evening meal						
Grilled salmon 120 g (4 oz)		4				
Steamed broccoli (2 florets) 3 tbsp carrots						2

	Carbs	Protein	Fat	Dairy	Fruit	Veg
Boiled new potatoes (240 g/ 8½ oz)	2					
Strawberries (80 g/3 oz)					1	
Supper						
3 rye crispbreads	1					
1 tbsp low-fat hummus		1				
10 olives			1			
Cup of herbal tea						
200 ml (7 fl oz) milk in tea and coffee during the day				1		
TOTAL IN DAY	7	9	4	3	2	5

Typical Non-Diet Day for Men

	2-Day Diet Portions					
Breakfast	Carbs	Protein	Fat	Dairy	Fruit	Veg
Bowl of porridge made with 40 g (1½ oz) porridge oats and 200 ml (7 fl oz) semi-skimmed milk. Cup of tea	2			1		
1 boiled egg		1				
Mid-morning						
Banana					1	
1 oatcake	1					
1 tsp peanut butter			1			
Celery sticks						1
Cup of coffee						
Lunch						
Tuna pasta salad						
60 g (2 oz) wholemeal pasta twists (dry weight)	2					

180 g (6 oz) tuna in spring water (drained weight)		4				
3 tbsp butter beans		2				
Bowl of lettuce, 10 cherry tomatoes, ¼ sliced pepper						3
1 tbsp of low-fat mayonnaise			1			
Fruit yoghurt (150 g/5 oz)				1		
Low-calorie drink/water						
Mid-afternoon						
Handful of pistachio nuts (15 g/½ oz)			2			
Cup of tea						
Evening meal						
Grilled salmon (120 g/ 4 oz)		4				
Steamed broccoli (2 florets) 3 tbsp carrots						2
Boiled new potatoes (240 g/ 8½ oz)	2					
½ corn on the cob	1					
Strawberries (80 g/3 oz)					1	
Supper						
3 rye crispbreads	1					
1 tbsp low-fat hummus		1				
10 olives			1			
Cup of herbal tea						
200 ml (7 fl oz) milk in tea and coffee during the day				1		
TOTAL IN DAY	9	12	5	3	2	6

Why exercise is important

Try to be as active as possible while doing The 2-Day Diet. Left to our own devices we tend to move less rather than more when we diet and research shows that our activity levels drop by around 40 per cent on average. When you move less you need fewer calories, making it harder to lose weight.[8] Regular exercise will speed up your weight loss, enhance the health benefits of The 2-Day Diet and boost your mood and energy levels.

▶ Exercise burns extra calories so helps combat the drop in your metabolic rate that occurs when you lose weight.

▶ Exercise helps maintain muscle, which burns more calories than fat.

▶ Although exercise alone won't shift much weight – the combination of diet and exercise really works.[9]

▶ Exercise boosts your mood and immunity and helps you sleep better.

▶ A single exercise session can lower blood pressure, increase insulin sensitivity and lower the levels of harmful fats in your blood for 24 to 48 hours.[10]

▶ Being active for 150 minutes a week (i.e. half an hour five days a week) reduces your risk of type 2 diabetes, cuts heart disease and stroke risk by 30 per cent and helps to protect against osteoporosis and arthritis.[11]

▶ Three to four hours' exercise a week can cut your risk of breast and colon cancer by 30 per cent.[12]

How much exercise?

▶ Aim to build up to at least 150 minutes' moderate (or 75 minutes' vigorous) exercise each week. Once you have managed this for 6 months, gradually build up to 300 minutes' moderate (or 150 minutes' vigorous) exercise each week.

▶ **Moderate exercise** includes walking (at 2½–4 mph or 4–6.5 kph), leisurely cycling or swimming, mowing the lawn, at a level where your heart rate is raised and you are slightly out of breath but can still hold a conversation.

▶ **Vigorous exercise** is fast walking (4½ mph or 7.25 kph) or jogging, playing squash or high-impact aerobics, exercise or chopping wood, at a level where it is difficult to maintain a conversation.

Always talk to your doctor before starting a new exercise programme, especially if you are not used to exercising or have any existing medical conditions that affect your heart, lungs, joints or balance.

For weight loss and optimum health you need to combine:

▶ **Cardiovascular (aerobic) exercise**, which includes exercise such as brisk walking, cycling or swimming that raises your heart rate and makes you feel warm and slightly out of breath. Cardiovascular exercise helps burn calories and improve your fitness.

And:

▶ **Resistance exercise**, using light weights or your own body weight to work your muscles, with regular stretching to help your flexibility. This kind of exercise will increase your muscle mass, help maintain healthy joints, keep your bones strong and improve your balance, reducing the risk of falls. Aim to include two or three 10-minute sessions of resistance exercise each week.

Visit the website (www.thetwodaydiet.co.uk) for more exercise information.

'I feel very alive especially doing The 2-Day Diet along with fitness routine every day. Even though I don't spend hours in the gym I feel so fit and healthy.' Alicia, 47

Why The 2-Day Diet works

Cutting down for two days is easier than cutting down every day

Most people in our trials found it easier to stick to two strict diet days rather than cut calories every day of the week. The 2-Day Diet is a huge relief after the grind of everyday dieting, which many had repeatedly tried to do. Our seven-day and 2-Day Dieters both started well, with 8 in 10 of them sticking to their diets during the first month. As time passed, the seven-day diet became more of a struggle. After three months,

70 per cent of 2-Day Dieters were still following their diet, compared to only 40 per cent of the seven-day group. 2-Day Dieters told us that they find the diet easier because it has clear rules and they could focus all their dieting efforts on two days. Research shows diets with clear rules and limited choice are easier to stick to than healthy-eating, low-calorie diets with flexible rules.[13]

Our bodies may even be biologically programmed for this type of 'intermittent' eating. The idea that we should have spells of restriction in between spells of normal intake isn't new. Some people argue that it's similar to our hunter-gatherer Palaeolithic ancestors, who frequently had periods with very little food, interspersed with spells of eating more, when food was available and abundant.

CASE STUDY: Mark

Mark, 37, lost two stone on The 2-Day Diet. His weight had crept up to 13 st 10 lbs after too many business lunches and an injury that stopped him exercising.

'This diet was so simple. You don't need to spend lots of time weighing and measuring, there's plenty of choice, you don't miss out on foods you like and so it doesn't really feel like you're on a diet. All diets are hard at first but after a few weeks the way you eat becomes a habit – the hardest thing was breakfast on diet days and bread, as that was one of my favourites.

'I usually did Monday and Tuesday. This made it easier as it was right after the weekend where you have probably had the odd treat and it gets them out of the way at the start of the week.'

You don't feel hungry on the diet

Not only did our dieters not complain of feeling hungry, they said they felt really healthy and energised on the diet days. In fact they felt so good that it made them want to do it again, week after week!

The 2-Day Diet retrains your eating habits

The 2-Day Diet gives you a break from your normal eating habits each week. This was a revelation to our dieters, many of whom became aware of what they ate for the first time, and better understood when and why they normally ate. This helped them to identify what triggered them to eat, and importantly to overeat. The 2-Day Diet helps you to take control of what you eat, which is the (often elusive) key to long-term success.

Although some people worry that they will overeat on the non-diet days, one of the most exciting and consistent findings of our research was that most people naturally restrict themselves on their non-diet days. On average our 2-Day Dieters ate about 25 per cent less than they normally would. This boosted their weight loss and meant that 2-Day Dieters lost even more weight than we expected!

'I found that it really helped to drink a lot, more than normal in fact, hot drinks, water and diet drinks as well'.
Sarah, 52

You will appreciate food more

Dramatically cutting calories for two days a week helps you to relearn how hunger feels and what a 'normal' serving looks like. You will learn to eat more slowly, appreciate smaller amounts and really enjoy your food both on your two diet and five non-diet days. This will help you to rediscover how much food you really need, rather than the amount you have become used to eating.

CASE STUDY: Pam

Pam, 41, has always struggled with her weight and has tried lots of diets but thanks to The 2-Day Diet she has gone from a size 22 to an 18 and the weight is still coming off.

'None of the other diets really suited me because they didn't let me enjoy the foods I like and not feel guilty about having a drink or two at the weekends. The 2-Day Diet has been great. My husband and I started it together and six months on I have slowly but surely lost just over a stone – I'm aiming for two more. Even after a two-week holiday I managed to keep most of the weight off and get right back into the diet afterwards. I feel so much fitter and less lethargic and actually want to do more exercise. And as this diet is only two days it's easier to get back into it if you have a blip. It has made me feel better in myself, more confident and fitter. I no longer suffer as much with knee problems or breathlessness.'

The 2-Day Diet boosts your dieting confidence

A daily diet can be daunting. By following The 2-Day Diet for just two days a week, you will discover that you really can resist temptation. We have found this boosts confidence in our dieters. Knowing you can master your diet and food cravings for two days can actually reinforce your desire to be in control of your diet on the other days of the week.

> *'I've tried so many diets in the past and failed that I
> didn't believe this one could be different. It was hard at
> first but it worked. I surprised myself that I could go two
> whole days without bread or biscuits – I feel that I'm back
> in control of my eating again.'* Michelle, 43

The 2-Day Diet helps you lose fat rather than calorie-burning muscle

The best diets target fat and preserve muscle. Muscle doesn't just make you look and feel more toned, it's also the key to effective calorie-burning. Even when your muscles are resting they burn up to seven times as many calories as fat.

There is inevitably some loss of muscle when we lose weight. Dieters who followed The 2-Day Diet found that they lost more fat and less muscle than the seven-day dieters and even more than if they had followed a daily very low-calorie diet (less than 800 kcal per day).

	2-Day Diet	7-Day Low Calorie Diet	7-Day Very Low Calorie Diet
How much of the weight loss was fat	80%	70%	60%
Fat lost for every stone (6.4 kg) of weight lost	5.1 kg (11. 2 lb)	4.5 kg (9.8 lb)	3.8 kg (8.4 lb)
Muscle lost for every stone (6.4 kg) of weight lost	1.3 kg (2.8 lb)	1.9 kg (4.2 lb)	2.6 kg (5.6 lb)

Because The 2-Day Diet promotes fat loss and minimises muscle loss, it should help to limit the dip in your metabolic rate that happens when we lose weight. The 2-Day Diet may also help burn a few more calories because of its high protein content – our bodies use 10 times more calories digesting and processing protein than for fat or carbohydrates. Although this only burns an extra 65–70 calories a day, when you're trying to lose weight every little helps.

The 2-Day Diet gives rapid results

Losing weight can feel like hard work, and there are no quick fixes. Fat-burning is a complex process and it's hard to lose more than 2 kg (4 lb) of fat a week. Rapid weight loss helps keep you on track and you won't need to spend weeks on The 2-Day Diet before you see a difference. The 2-Day Diet performs better than seven-day dieting right from the start. Our dieters lost fat about one and a half times more quickly on The 2-Day Diet than those on the conventional seven-day diet and, crucially, kept the weight off longer term. When we have caught up with 2-Day Dieters after 12–15 months they had lost on average 1–1½ stone and maintained their beneficial reductions in blood pressure, cholesterol and insulin.

Key points

▶ The 2-Day Diet is a new, clinically proven, nutritionally balanced approach for weight loss, designed to maximise weight loss and preserve calorie-burning muscle.

▶ The 2-Day Diet involves eating protein, healthy fats, fruit and vegetables for two consecutive days each week and a balanced, Mediterranean-style diet for the remaining five days.

▶ Published research shows that The 2-Day Diet achieves better and more rapid weight loss plus greater health benefits than a standard daily low-calorie diet.

▶ Many 2-Day Dieters view it as a lifestyle change – not a diet.

▶ Our 2-Day Dieters have retrained their eating habits and kept their weight off long term.

Making it work

The 2-Day Diet is about eating the right type and amounts of food, which inevitably means making changes. This isn't always easy, but being committed, motivated and prepared is vital to your weight-loss success.

Step 1: Prepare yourself for the challenge ahead

In the early days you will need to invest a bit of time, commitment and planning and getting to grips with the food types and amounts you can eat on your two diet days. For some people this could be a big change, but don't be put off. It is definitely time well spent. The message from our 2-Day Dieters was that although making the changes took some effort at first, the diet days rapidly became second nature and the longer they stuck to it, the easier it got. This is in stark contrast to many other diets which seem to get harder as you go on.

'You have to spend the first couple of weeks getting used to the diet, but the longer you stick with it – the easier it gets!' Linda, 31

Step 2: Build your support system

Ask friends and family for support and, if you can, find someone to do the diet with you. Make sure other people know that you're trying to lose weight and would prefer not to be given sweets or chocolates as gifts. We know that many couples have done The 2-Day Diet together and have supported and motivated each other throughout.

'Make sure you have full support from the rest of your family so they don't try and offer you things you're not supposed to have and can help you on those days you are tempted.' Mark, 37

Visit www.thetwodaydiet.co.uk for further information, support and tips or find us on Facebook to connect with other 2-Day Dieters and to share your experiences.

Step 3: Set your weight-loss goals
Be ambitious but realistic

Everyone wants to shed weight as quickly as possible and if you stick to The 2-Day Diet you will achieve successful, rapid weight loss. Many of our dieters lost more weight than they expected. They also lost it about 50 per cent faster than those on an every day diet. Remember that most people won't lose any more than 2 kg (4 lb) of fat per week. Any other weight loss is likely to be due to loss of water. The table below gives you some idea of how quickly our 2-Day Dieters lost weight and inches – and how quickly they made improvements to their blood pressure, cholesterol and insulin levels. If you follow The 2-Day Diet correctly, most of the weight you lose will be fat and, crucially, you should lose a substantial amount of that dangerous fat stored around your waist and vital organs.

	Month 1 (average)	Month 1 (maximum)	Over 3 months (average)	Over 3 months (maximum)
Weight loss	2.7 kg (6 lb)	6.6 kg (14½ lb)	5.8 kg (13 lb)	14.5 kg (32 lb)
Fat loss	2 kg (4½ lb)	5 kg (11 lb)	4.5 kg (10 lb)	11 kg (24 lb)
Drop in waist size	2.6 cm (1 in)	6 cm (2⅓ in)	6 cm (2⅓ in)	19 cm (7½ in)
Insulin % drop	10%	74%	12%	76%
Cholesterol % drop	6%	34%	6%	34%
Blood pressure % drop	11%	38%	11%	40%

'I wanted to do the diet as I'd put on the usual extra weight over Christmas. I ended up losing these pounds easily and a few more besides – 11 lbs in total.' Karen, 45

What is your weight-loss goal?

Although losing 5–10 per cent of your weight (e.g. if you weigh 11 stone and aim to get down to 10–10½ stone) might not sound much, it is enough to give you instant health benefits, including cutting the risk of type 2 diabetes[14] (by 60 per cent),[12] heart disease (by 50–60 per cent)[15] and breast cancer (by 25–40 per cent).[2]

It's up to you to decide how much you want to lose. Don't be scared to be ambitious, as long as your goal is realistic and achievable. It may help to break your goals into two- or three-month blocks to boost your confidence and motivation.

Step 4: Plan ahead

If you have the right foods at home and work you're more likely to succeed. On diet days have a healthy homemade lunch and snacks with you at work so you don't have to resort to high-carb foods in the canteen or sandwich shop. Late afternoon and evening are typical danger times for snacking but you can find a list of 2-Day Diet snacks on page 12. Make sure you have everything you need for your evening meal ahead of time so you're not tempted to pick up other food in the supermarket.

> *'I plan two days in advance with The 2-Day Diet portions, especially protein, and this helps a lot.'*
> *Annie, 34*

> *'If I make soup I make a big batch and freeze it in portions ready for the following weeks.' Sarah, 49*

'I always have eggs in the cupboard as they're quick, easy and tasty if you're short on time.' Louise, 55

Step 5: Watch your portion sizes

One of the reasons many of us struggle with our weight is that our servings are too big. Twenty years ago a medium-sized slice of bread weighed 30 g (1 oz) and contained 65 calories; today it weighs 45 g (1½ oz) and contains 90 calories. That's why, as well as showing you the types of food to eat, The 2-Day Diet provides clear guidelines on the amounts to eat on your diet days and non-diet days for dieting success.

Portion sizes should not be an issue on the two diet days when the balance of foods means that you tend to self-limit what you eat. We certainly don't expect you to weigh all your foods – we provide simple guidelines for gauging portion sizes alongside the weights of food on both the two diet days and the other five days. On non-diet days some of our dieters find it helpful to weigh foods such as breakfast cereals, pasta and rice, which are easy to overdo, until they got used to the recommended serving sizes.

Track your portions

For the first few weeks use The 2-Day Diet Tracker (see page 18 and visit www.thetwodaydiet.co.uk) to record what you've eaten and make sure you are on track with the diet.

Step 6: Watch your liquid calories

It's important that you have plenty to drink on both diet and non-diet days. Often we eat when we are actually thirsty. Drinking before or with a meal can make us feel fuller, so we don't eat so much, but choose wisely. Some drinks are calorie loaded and these fluid calories bypass normal appetite controls making it easy to consume too many. A large full-fat milk latte comes in at a whopping 223 calories and even the skimmed-milk version contains 131 calories. By contrast an americano with semi-skimmed milk contains only 20 calories, so drink coffee or tea with a splash of milk or herbal teas instead.

Step 7: Sit at a table to eat

Eating on the run, while watching TV, sitting at your desk, or even listening to the radio, means that your focus is elsewhere and you will tend to consume more calories – simply because you don't notice what or how much you are eating. In one study people eating crisps while watching TV ate around 40 per cent more than on another occasion when they didn't watch any TV.[16]

To avoid uncontrolled munching, sit down at a table, eat slowly and savour each mouthful. It takes about 15 minutes for your brain to let your stomach know that you have eaten enough, so make yourself wait after finishing a meal to decide whether you really need seconds or dessert.

'Dieting on the two days was much easier than I had expected. I also found that I was much more mindful of my eating over the five normal eating days – I didn't want to undo all that good work!' Lizzie, 24

Step 8: Don't fall into the diet food trap

The supermarkets are full of them – the low-fat, low-sugar 'diet' foods that promise an easy way to eat fewer calories and lose weight. The 2-Day Diet is mainly based on unprocessed foods. The only 'diet' foods that may be useful are low-fat foods like low-fat mayonnaise, low-fat cheese and those that use artificial sweeteners with no added sugar, such as diet drinks.

*'It's quite normal to crave carbs on your two diet days at
first but I found that it gets easier every week so persevere.'*
Steve, 47

Step 9: Monitor your progress

We know that dieters who monitor themselves do better. The
way you feel in your clothes is one indicator, but we recommend you weigh yourself and measure your waist and hips once
a week. Weigh yourself at the same time of day, ideally in the
morning, without clothes or shoes, using the same scales, and
make a note of the results. Remember that, for women, weight
and waist measurements are often greater just before your
period because of fluid retention. Because you lose water on
the two diet days of The 2-Day Diet you will get a more accurate measure if you weigh yourself immediately before rather
than after your diet days each week. If you step on the scales
immediately after the two days you will be lighter as you will
have lost fluid as well as some fat.

Key points

▶ Do your groundwork. Calculate your Body Mass Index,
and work out your body fat level so you know how much
weight you need to lose. You can find a BMI calculator and
Body Fat Ready Reckoner at www.thetwodaydiet.co.uk.

▶ Set yourself clear short-term and long-term weight-loss
goals so that you know what you are aiming for.

▶ Make sure you know exactly what the diet involves and
you are well prepared in advance and make a plan.

▶ Invest a bit of time up front and it will pay back dividends.

How to keep the weight off

Once you've reached your target weight you want to avoid regaining it. We know all too well that keeping weight off is a new challenge that requires you to keep your calorie intake down and exercise levels up and not slip back into old habits.

To keep weight off you need to keep to the principles of The 2-Day Diet but switch to The 1-Day Maintenance Diet (having one diet day per week rather than two) and keep your activity levels up. You will find that 1-Day Maintenance is easy to do and although we call it a diet, it's really just a way of life. Our dieters said it became second nature to them and our research showed that our 2-Day Dieters who moved on to the Maintenance Diet, not only succeeded in keeping the weight off, they also maintained the beneficial reductions in their blood pressure, cholesterol and insulin. Normally, when you stop following a standard calorie-controlled diet and revert to eating normally every day you lose some of the health benefits you've gained from losing weight, particularly the drop in insulin, blood pressure and cholesterol.

Meeting the new challenge

To keep the weight off permanently you need to adjust your mental approach. You don't have the excitement of a new diet and no one will congratulate you on keeping the weight off (although they should!) It is a challenge, but many of our dieters have managed to make weight control a way of life using the expertise they have gained from following The 2-Day Diet.

The 1-Day Maintenance Diet

The 1-Day Maintenance Diet is based on The 2-Day Diet, but instead of two diet days each week you now only have to do one. For the rest of the week (the other six days) we advise you to eat the healthy Mediterranean diet you have followed with The 2-Day Diet. Like The 2-Day Diet, you should not have to count calories or weigh food but make sure that you are keeping within the recommended amounts of 2-Day Diet portions (see Ready Reckoners for weight-loss maintenance on page 164). As before, have plenty of healthy protein foods, fibre and vegetables.

'Because it's only one day I find it easy to do – everyone can be "good" one day a week! It doesn't really impact on my lifestyle and I can adjust it to suit times like holidays and Christmas.' Jane, 51

Getting used to the new you

Your body changes when you lose weight. Because you weigh less, you need fewer calories to function than you did before you started The 2-Day Diet.

Dieting may mean that your muscles will have become more efficient and need less energy to function. While this is good news for your muscles, it means that you could now need up to 15 per cent fewer calories than someone of the same weight who hasn't dieted.

So, having lost your weight you now need to eat around 400 to 600 fewer calories each day than you did before you started. You can see why you also need to keep exercising to help burn off calories and offset the drop in your metabolic rate.[17]

How to keep the weight off

Step 1: Monitor yourself and take immediate action if your weight starts creeping up

Keeping a close eye on your weight is a key part of keeping the weight off. If you spot weight gain early you can act quickly, and reverse the trend. It's relatively easy to shed a few extra pounds but when that turns into half a stone it becomes far more difficult. Try to weigh yourself weekly as well as keeping an eye on how your clothes fit. Don't be tempted to 'cheat' by always wearing joggers or leggings; fitted clothes are better indicators.

Weight can fluctuate by 1–2 kg (2–4 lb) depending on the time of day or time of cycle for premenopausal women. Try to weigh yourself first thing in the morning. If you have gained just a pound or two, watch your diet and increase your exercise over the next few weeks. Any more than this and you should go back on to your 2-Day regime until you have lost the extra weight – and then go back to the 1-Day Maintenance Plan again.

> *'Once I reached my goal weight I do one day per week to keep me in check. I usually gain about 4 lb (1.8 kg) when I go on holiday. Now I just go back on to two days per week when I get home and it comes back off.'* Annabell, 35

Step 2: Find support

Positive comments and support from your nearest and dearest are great motivators. Ask the people who supported you when you were dieting to keep encouraging you as you work at keeping it off.

Getting peer support from other maintainers who are also trying to keep the weight off can be enormously helpful. Visit our website www.thetwodaydiet.co.uk or find us on Facebook, for support and ideas from other maintainers.

Step 3: Watch for portion creep

Since following The 2-Day Diet you should have a far more realistic idea about healthy portion sizes, but it's still important to keep track as it's surprisingly easy for portions to grow. Don't go back to just pouring out cereal, rice or pasta – use spoons or a small cup for measuring. It might also help to use smaller plates and bowls and small cutlery. At the end of the day tot up the number of food portions you have had against the recommended amounts for the diet – you can find a 2-Day Diet tracker at www.thetwodaydiet.co.uk.

Step 4: Stay active

We have also designed an exercise plan to help you keep the weight off (see www.thetwodaydiet.co.uk). Try to be as active as possible. You should aim to do 300 minutes' moderate (or 150 minutes' vigorous) exercise spread over the week. Again, it can be easy to let this slip, so monitor what you do. We know that successful maintainers keep a close eye on their activity levels as well as their weight. You can do a quick mental tally of how active you have been at the end of each day. Write it in a diary or use The 2-Day Diet online tool.

Step 5: Be prepared for danger times

Use the strategies you have learnt while doing the diet to fend off temptation and deal with difficult situations. You might decide to allow yourself to eat more freely at particular social events, but compensate by eating less in the days before and afterwards. If there are times when you have lapsed, don't give up; instead, learn from them to enable you to cope better the next time around.

Step 6: Stay motivated

Remind yourself why you wanted to lose weight and of how far you have come – before and after pictures are a great record of your success. Set yourself targets to keep the weight off, for example aiming for a forthcoming event such as a holiday, party or wedding. Reward yourself as much for keeping the weight off as for losing it in the first place. Plan a non-food treat for the end of each month that you keep your weight off.

Step 7: Keep it varied

Building good diet and exercise habits can be the key to your weight-loss success but if you feel that you're in a rut, ring the changes. Try different foods and experiment with other recipes in this book or *The 2-Day Diet Cookbook*. Set yourself new exercise goals, introduce a different activity to your weekly routine or take up a new challenge such as a half marathon or a charity bike ride.

Key points

▶ Once you have lost weight your body needs fewer calories to function. The tried-and-tested 1-Day Maintenance Diet is designed to ensure that you keep the weight off.

▶ The 1-Day Maintenance Diet involves doing one diet day every week, six days of a Mediterranean diet and being as active as possible.

▶ Key elements of successful maintenance are regularly monitoring your weight and serving sizes, staying active, setting a new goal and reward system for yourself, and getting the support you need.

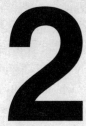

2
Your Questions Answered

In this chapter we have tried to answer the questions you may have about The 2-Day Diet and how it works. Dieting for just two days a week is such a different approach to weight loss that people often worry whether they are doing it correctly and how it will affect their body and health. In this chapter we've tried to address all these issues and more.

Although people have lots of questions, our research, and the feedback we've received from many dieters, suggests that most were pleasantly surprised by how easy they found the diet and actually enjoyed this new, healthier way of eating. The fact that it's simple but structured helps you to adapt quickly and develop a routine. While most diets get harder to stick to over time, you will find The 2-Day Diet gets easier the longer you are on it and will help you to permanently change your eating habits. The two diet days help you to practise eating healthier foods and smaller portions, learn to recognise 'real' hunger again and enjoy and savour your food. In short, The 2–Day Diet puts you back in control of your eating.

The diet is particularly easy to fit into family life and meal-times and means that the whole family eats more healthily. On your diet days the rest of the family can eat the same meals, but with added carbohydrate foods, such as potatoes, rice or pasta. For the five non-diet days the whole family will benefit from healthy Mediterranean eating.

The diet works just as well for men as for women. Although most of our original research was with women, The 2-Day Diet has inspired many men who would never have considered dieting to start losing weight. We've also heard of lots of couples who have successfully done the diet together. As well as helping them both to lose weight they have found it enjoyable and have been able to support and encourage each other through the process.

CASE STUDY: George and Oxana

George and Oxana decided to do the diet together which helped to make it work. George, 46, has lost five stone while Oxana, 44, has achieved her goal of dropping a dress size.

'George is a great encouragement – even to the point of gentle acts of persuasion when I slip up! And when I encourage him, I'm also encouraging myself," says Oxana. And for George, who has never dieted before, the whole process has been a revelation. 'I have always avoided dieting but following The 2-Day Diet together has made it so much easier, because we can then plan, shop, cook, and encourage each other in times of weakness, and we also reap the rewards together as a couple, and one of the rewards is dining out, little treats, and general state of wellbeing that we are a Team.'

About the diet

Why two days?

We wanted to get away from the grind of everyday dieting, which we know people struggle with. We chose two days as we thought this would be achievable, would reduce overall calorie intake enough for weight loss, and long enough to retrain eating habits.

Some people worry that The 2-Day Diet is a type of yo-yo dieting whereby you lose weight for two days each week and rebound back in between. In fact there is no yo-yoing on The 2-Day Diet. By doing the two diet days every week and following a healthy diet in between, your weight will steadily drop while following the plan.

How is this different from other 5:2 diets?

On The 2-Day Diet you don't need to count calories, skip meals or go hungry. This is not a fasting diet and you shouldn't feel deprived. On your two diet days, you simply need to avoid carbohydrates and sugars. You can still eat plenty of protein, healthy fats, dairy, low-carb fruit and vegetables. On the non-diet days of the week you eat a normal healthy diet. Unlike other 5:2 diets, The 2-Day Diet has been extensively researched, tested on real-life dieters and proven to work in clinical trials. The diet has been designed by a dietitian to keep you feeling full, maximise the amount of fat you lose and preserve your calorie-burning muscle. The 2-Day Diet is nutritionally complete so there is no need to take supplements. We have also included guidelines on what to eat on the other non-diet days, suggesting maximum amounts because we know that weight loss and the health benefits of this type of diet can only be achieved if you don't overeat on the other five days.

Do I have to diet for two consecutive days?

We recommend doing the two days together because our research found that most dieters find the second consecutive day as easy or easier than the first as they are used to eating less. Doing the two days together also helps ensure that you get round to doing the second day. Two diet days back to back may also have additional health benefits because this provides a prolonged period when the body has a lower calorie intake and your body cells are not being 'overfed'. We recommend that you follow the diet for two whole days – so start your diet day with breakfast on Day 1 and include supper on Day 2. You will revert to normal eating at breakfast the morning after. This gives your body 60 hours when it is getting reduced calories and is in a healthier metabolic state when cells are not overfed and can divert their efforts from growing to repairing damage. By contrast, many 5:2 diets suggest just two 24-hour restrictions from 10pm one day until 10pm the next. If you consider the fact that you don't eat overnight (so you always have a 12-hour fast anyway) these diets only restrict your calorie intake for an additional 12 hours, which may not be long enough to bring about the metabolic changes that are so beneficial to health.

If you struggle to do the two days together, doing them separately is fine (as long as you do them both!) In our research the 5 per cent of our dieters who often did their two days separately still managed to lose weight.

*'I had never successfully dieted and kept weight off before
I tried The 2-Day Diet. In fact I have always regained
the weight and then usually extra too. The 2-Day Diet is
different – it's a lifestyle change I can actually live with.'*
Marie, 33

Can I do more than two diet days to speed up my weight loss?

We don't recommend doing more than two diet days per week because the whole diet (that is to say the two diet days and the five non-diet days) has been balanced to ensure that all your nutritional requirements are met. You will achieve good weight loss with two diet days each week.

Aren't the diet days just the same as an Atkins- or Dukan-style diet?

The 2-Day Diet days are low-carb and so have some similarities to low-carb, high-protein diets such as Atkins or Dukan, but this diet is different. While the low-carb days are designed for weight loss, they are also designed for optimum health, ensuring that you get the right balance of healthy fats (which are low in saturates, high in monounsaturates and omega-3 fats) and fruit and vegetables. And because you are only doing low-carb for two days and eating a healthy, balanced diet for the rest of the week, this diet is very different.

Can I still do the diet if I am a healthy weight?

The first thing is to check that you *are* a healthy weight with a healthy level of body fat (see page 4). One in four people who have a healthy weight on the scales may have too much fat around their waist, increasing their risk of heart disease, type

2 diabetes and possibly certain cancers. If this sounds like you, then losing weight would be beneficial for your health. If you have a healthy weight and waist measurement, two-day dieting is probably not a good idea as we don't know the impact of the diet on healthy-weight individuals. However, doing one diet day a week (see page 40) will help to keep your weight stable, especially if you are at a stage of your life when you might be particularly vulnerable to weight gain.

We do not recommend doing either one or two days of the diet if you are underweight (BMI < 18.5 – see BMI calculator at www.thetwodaydiet.co.uk) because lighter people have less body fat (which protects us from losing muscle when we diet) and stand to lose muscle mass.

Is the diet suitable for vegetarians?

The diet works just as well for vegetarians as for meat and fish eaters. You can find details of the vegetarian 2-Day Diet in Appendix A at the back of the book (see page 145). The key is to ensure that you include enough protein and don't overload on carbs – there are plenty of filling vegetarian protein foods and we've included lots of tasty vegetarian recipes (see pages 86, 121) for your two diet days and the rest of the week.

Is the diet better suited to men than women?

We are often asked whether The 2-Day Diet is safe for women and if it can affect fertility. Most of our research has been in women and our 2-Day Dieters still had regular menstrual cycles. However, we would not advocate The 2-Day Diet for women who are planning to become pregnant in the very near future. If you need to lose weight it's advisable to do this before you conceive and not at the time of conception or during pregnancy itself. Our 2-Day Diet is no exception and should not be undertaken during these times.

Making it work

How should I plan my diet days?

Choose which days of the week work best for you. Many of our dieters opt for busy work days when they don't have time to think about missing food, whereas others prefer to do them at the weekend when there's more time to be organised. Whichever days you choose, try, if possible, to keep to the same days each week to establish a habit. However, the beauty of only having to diet for two days is that you can swap your days, if necessary, to fit into your week's schedule.

I've heard that 8-hour diets, where you just eat for a few hours in the middle of the day, can work just as well.

What matters for weight loss is the total calories you have in a day. If just eating in the middle of the day means you have fewer calories overall then you will lose weight. There is little research into the weight loss or health benefits of this pattern of eating. The most rigorous study compared eating the same amount of food in a four-hour window to having three meals throughout the day and failed to show obvious weight loss or health benefits. Those who ate their food in a four-hour window ended up being marginally lighter as they had a slightly lower calorie intake. Despite this they had a slightly higher blood pressure and levels of fat in their blood and poorer insulin function, suggesting that this pattern of eating was not beneficial and perhaps may not be suited to our metabolism.[1]

CASE STUDY: Katrina

Katrina, 42, started The 2-Day Diet after she gained weight over Christmas.

'I chose to have my diet days at the beginning of the week and must admit the first week I found breakfast a challenge because I'm so used to having either toast or cereal. The first week I had fruit and a yoghurt for breakfast but that felt quite restrictive – getting my head round the idea that I could have bacon/eggs or an omelette made it so much easier.

'I have done slimming clubs in the past and lost weight but The 2-Day Diet is so much easier. I've also felt far less hungry than I did on the other diets. And I like the fact that it's flexible – if I have weeks where I'm out a lot and it's not easy to avoid carbs, I switch my days that week or – as when I was away from home for a long period on business – I switch to a one day a week maintenance plan.'

Is it better to have lots of small meals throughout the day rather than a few large meals?

Some people argue that eating frequently helps to control your appetite because it stops you getting really hungry and then overeating at mealtimes. Others say that constant snacking just encourages you to focus on food and makes you eat more. There is no evidence that frequent eating is better for controlling hunger or reducing levels of 'appetite' hormones. And there is no difference in your metabolic rate whether you eat two large meals, or six or seven smaller ones a day if you consume the same amount overall.[2] The bottom line is not how often you eat, but how much you eat in total within a day. You probably know the pattern of eating that suits you best and helps control your appetite. If not, experiment with it and see whether it works better for you to stick with two or three large meals, or to have five or six smaller ones.

Isn't it better to eat early in the day, because eating after 5pm is more fattening?

Lots of people believe that eating in the evening makes you put on weight, but research shows that it's the total number of calories you consume over the 24 hours that determines whether you gain or lose weight. Food eaten in the evening is no more likely to be stored as fat than food eaten earlier in the day.[3]

Be aware of when you overeat and what triggers the over-eating. If you get the munchies in the evenings or find it hard not to eat a large evening meal even if you aren't hungry, watch out for these times. Evenings are danger times for many people, especially if they are watching TV. It helps to stay busy, so do the ironing or something practical with your hands (such as knitting) while watching TV. If you need something, have a hot drink. It also helps to brush your teeth after the last time you eat – to signal to your body that eating is over for the day.

Do I have to eat breakfast?

Breakfast is often quoted as a vital meal for dieters as it kick-starts your metabolism and helps stop overeating later in the day. Evidence suggests you should not force yourself to eat breakfast if you don't want it. Some of us are 'morning' people, who need breakfast to get going, but if you can't face breakfast first thing, wait until you are hungry. When researchers from Roehampton University asked people who didn't normally eat breakfast to include it, they didn't eat less for the rest of the day – they ate 300 calories more than normal. But when people who always ate breakfast were asked to skip it, they overate later in the day.[4] In other words we are probably all wired differently, so do whatever works for you.

> *'I've never been a breakfast person so I skip it and eat later. My advice is don't be a slave to your normal mealtimes on diet days – if it works better for you break your normal habits and eat when you're hungry.' Jan, 37*

Can I have snacks?

If you can't get through to lunch without a snack mid-morning then go ahead! Choose from one of the healthy snack ideas you'll find on page 12. If you don't need to snack, just stick with your three meals a day. Don't forget that snacks count towards your total food allowance on the two diet days.

I'm worried about bingeing on non-diet days – am I likely to overeat?

It's an understandable concern. However, we have consistently found that our 2-Day Dieters didn't want to binge on their non-diet days, they actually wanted to eat less. A key feature of The 2-Day Diet is that it appears to reset your appetite and retrain your eating behaviour for the whole week. Our dieters naturally ended up eating 25 per cent less than normal on non-diet days.

Do I have to follow the diet – can't I just cut calories?

We don't advise going without food or devising your own reduced-calorie diet. This Diet has been developed by a research dietitian and is designed to have the optimum balance of foods to keep you feeling full, cover your nutritional requirements, burn fat and preserve muscle mass, which is key to maintaining your metabolic rate and long-term weight-loss success. If you invent your own low-calorie diet you run the risk of it not being nutritionally complete, being hungrier than you need to be, which makes it difficult to adhere to, and it won't necessarily target fat and preserve muscle mass.

'I like this diet because it looks and feels more healthy than just counting calories. Because I'm eating good food, I feel more nourished.' Liam, 59

Can I exercise on my diet days?

Lots of people think that because they are limiting calories, and particularly carbs, they won't have the energy to exercise on diet days. In fact our dieters were just as likely to exercise on these days as the non-diet days and the calorie and carb restrictions didn't reduce their ability to exercise or increase their levels of fatigue – a finding backed up by other research.[5] This research suggests that if you exercise while following a low-carb, low-calorie diet you might burn more fat. On diet days make sure you stay well hydrated and get enough sodium, potassium and permitted carbohydrates by having your dairy, fruit and vegetable allowance.

If you are normally a vigorous exerciser and are struggling with this on diet days, try replacing vigorous with moderate activity and save the vigorous workouts for your non-diet days.

'I thought it would be hard to exercise on diet days but I had far more energy than I expected.' June, 43

How to eat on diet days

Do I need to take a vitamin supplement?

You don't need to take a supplement on this diet because it is designed to ensure that you get all the nutrients you need. It's always better to get nutrients from food because this provides a gradual supply of nutrients that are more easily absorbed by your body than the one-off dose delivered in a supplement. When you go on any diet and eat less, you often reduce your intake of vitamins and minerals, particularly calcium, iron, zinc and magnesium and we find many of our dieters already have low intakes of selenium, folate and vitamin A. Good sources of these important nutrients on diet days are:

Calcium: from low-fat dairy foods, calcium-fortified soya, almonds, eggs, beans, leafy green vegetables, tinned oily fish (if you eat the bones), tofu with added calcium.

Iron: from lean meat, eggs, green vegetables, nuts.

Zinc: from shellfish, Quorn, lean meat, poultry, milk, eggs, nuts, cheese.

Magnesium: from fish, shellfish, Quorn, lean meat, leafy green vegetables, avocado, milk, nuts.

Selenium: from fish, shellfish, meat, Brazil nuts, eggs, mushrooms.

Folate: from liver, leafy green vegetables, fish, avocado.

Vitamin A: from herring, kipper, salmon, liver, eggs, fortified low-fat margarines or spreads.

Should I be eating nuts – aren't they very high in calories?

Although nuts are high in fat and calories they are packed with healthy monounsaturated and polyunsaturated omega-3 fats and polyphenols. Because they are also high in protein, they are very filling. Nuts may even help reduce the risk of stroke because they contain l-arginine, a substance that may make your artery walls more flexible and less prone to blood clots. A recent large Spanish study found that those who ate 25 g (1 oz) of nuts each day had 40 per cent less strokes than those who didn't.[6]

Eat unsalted nuts to keep your salt intake down, except if you are using nuts as a salty food on diet days (see the information on salt on page 14).

Can I include protein shakes?

Protein is particularly important as it stops you feeling hungry and helps maintain calorie-burning muscle. We recommend real protein food rather than shakes, which may be high in sugar and carbs. If you want to have a high-protein drink instead of food it's healthier (and cheaper) to make yourself a fruit smoothie (try the Papaya and golden linseed smoothie, page 76).

I'm dairy-free – can I still do the diet?

If you don't eat dairy foods you can replace your dairy portions with the equivalent quantities of calcium-fortified soya milk, yoghurts or an unsweetened nut milk. You can use rice or oat milk on non-diet days, but not on diet days as they are too high in carbs.

If you don't want to use a milk alternative, replace milk with more vegetable protein foods (see Appendix A, page 138).

Make sure you have plenty of non-dairy calcium from almonds, eggs, beans and leafy green vegetables, tinned oily fish (if you eat the bones) and tofu with added calcium.

I thought that diet fizzy drinks were bad for you – why are they allowed on this diet?

Sugary, fizzy drinks, which are loaded with sucrose and fructose, are very definitely not a part of The 2-Day Diet. The calories in these sugary drinks are directly converted to fat, which builds up in the liver. Some people *have* been surprised by the fact that we allow limited amounts of diet or low-calorie fizzy drinks containing artificial sweeteners. A recent study raised concerns that both sugary drinks and those containing the artificial sweetener aspartame may be linked with certain blood cancers. However, these were preliminary studies – one of them on animals – and there's not yet convincing evidence that sweeteners have adverse health effects. In an ideal world you would avoid sugar and artificial sweeteners, but if you do enjoy fizzy drinks we advise you to limit your intake to a maximum of 3 litres (nine cans) of diet drinks a week.

Is it okay to have plenty of tea and coffee on diet days?

Lots of people assume that too much caffeine (in tea and coffee) is bad for our health but there's little evidence for this. Both can be really useful on diet days providing a satisfying drink that fends off the urge to eat. Experts agree that for most people caffeine is not the cause of high blood pressure or risk of heart disease.[7] Tea and coffee contain disease-fighting antioxidants that could actually lower your risk of heart disease and certain cancers.

Can I have more vegetables and fruit than it says on the plan?

It is important to keep to just five portions of lower-carbohydrate vegetables on the diet days to ensure that the diet is low enough in carbs for maximum effect. You can swap the portion of fruit for two additional vegetable portions on these days, so you could have seven portions of low-carb vegetables on a diet day as well as the protein, dairy and fat portions.

On non-diet days we encourage at least five 80 g (3 oz) servings per day, but you can eat as many vegetables as you wish on these days. Don't have unlimited potatoes, beans or pulses on non-diet days as they count as carbohydrate and protein foods within the diet plan and would quickly push up your overall calorie intake.

Keep fruit within the suggested amounts as it is quite easy to over-consume on calories and carbohydrates from fruits.

Can I use sauces, spreads, honey or jam?

Flavouring your food with condiments, sauces and spreads helps make food more interesting and keeps you on track with your diet, but many are high in salt and sugar, and therefore calories.

On your diet days you can use mustard, horseradish sauce, yeast extract and mayonnaise. Other sauces and spreads are fine to use in small amounts on the non-diet days. Go for low-salt versions and only use small amounts of sweet pickles, chutneys and ready-made cranberry or apple sauce and redcurrant jelly, which can be quite high in sugar, calories and salt.

We suggest you use low-sugar jams or marmalade or pure fruit spreads. If you want to have honey (used in some 2-Day Diet recipes) a few tablespoons per week would count as one of your treat foods. See page 13 and Appendix A on page 144 for further information on flavourings.

I have a lot of weight to lose – is it possible to do this diet for a long time?

The great thing about The 2-Day Diet is that people can stick with it long term. When you reach your goal weight, switch to the 1-Day Maintenance Plan to keep the weight off. We have had people on The 2-Day Diet for up to two years and not seen any harmful effects.

How will I feel doing The 2-Day Diet?

Will I be hungry on my diet days?

You should not feel any hungrier on your two diet days than you did before you started the diet. We assessed 'hungriness' in our dieters both before they started the diet and while they were doing it and found that their 'hungriness' was exactly the same on their diet and non-diet days as it was pre-diet. It's easy to mistake hunger for thirst, so if you feel hungry have a drink and see if that helps. On diet days, make sure you have enough protein foods, nuts and dairy foods, which are particularly good at filling you up. If you feel hungry in the first few weeks of the diet, stick with it as most of our dieters found that it got easier as they got used to it.

'I have some peanuts or peanut butter and celery at 11am–noon. It fills you up and you don't need lunch till 2–3pm.' Jan, 29

CASE STUDY: James

James, 48, had never dieted before when he decided to embark on The 2-Day Diet, but he has managed to lose 1½ stone.

'When I started the diet I was the heaviest I had ever been and starting to feel unhealthy. I knew a few people who had done the diet and lost weight and most importantly I could see myself sticking to it – because it is only two days per week, you don't have to think about it all the time or always be thinking "I can't eat that".

'The hardest time for me was always mid-afternoon when I am hungry and there are biscuits at work, but it has been really easy to fit into my life. I do Mondays and Tuesdays, which are really busy days and I am thinking about other things. I tend to go for soups in the evening on diet days as they really fill you up. It's helped me feel much healthier and more energetic – I run and losing weight has made me much more likely to go out running than before.'

Why am I passing more water?

You will probably go to the toilet more often on diet days for two main reasons. Firstly, you will be mobilising glycogen, the carbohydrate stored in your muscles and liver. Glycogen releases water that your body then needs to get rid of. Secondly, burning fat increases the levels of ketones in the blood, which acts as a diuretic, making you want to use the toilet more often.

Ketones are a natural by-product of fat burning. They are not harmful unless they build up to extremely high levels, which won't happen on this diet. Ketones have a bad press as levels achieved with some daily very low-carbohydrate diets can lead to side effects including headache, nausea and bad breath. Our dieters typically doubled their level of ketones, but these levels are far lower than dieters on a longer-term very low-carbohydrate diet who experience five-fold increases in ketones.

> *'I find that I'm thirstier than usual on the diet days,*
> *so I always make sure I have a bottle of water to hand.'*
> *Anna, 27*

Will I feel more tired on my diet days?

Quite the contrary, most of our dieters felt good. Many reported feeling invigorated, cleansed and detoxed after diet days, which made them more committed to the diet and eating healthily for the rest of the week. They felt less bloated, less sluggish and more energetic and when we assessed their general mood and wellbeing, in most cases their mood improved and levels of tension, depression, anger, fatigue and confusion were halved.

Interestingly our dieters said that the two diet days each week feel like the first few days of a normal diet, with all the positive feelings of increased energy and sense of achievement that go with it. Revisiting those feelings every week gave them a boost and reinforced their motivation.

> *'The big thing for me is that this diet is achievable,*
> *maintainable and helps keep the weight off by offering*
> *a whole new healthier way of eating, with the odd treat*
> *allowed!' Pam, 43*

Will I have any side effects?

None of our dieters reported major problems although a few experienced headaches. If this happens, make sure you are drinking plenty (2 litres/4 pints) a day is usually enough. If you drink more than that, ensure you are including enough electrolytes (potassium, sodium and magnesium) from fruit, vegetables, dairy and protein foods, and you may need to include a salty food or drink on your diet days (see the information on salt on page 14). Although you don't have to cut down on tea and coffee, if you have done your headaches may be related to caffeine withdrawal. The drop in carbohydrate intake can also cause headaches but should improve as your body adjusts. A few people became constipated – if this happens make sure you get enough fluid and your full fruit and vegetable allowance on diet days with plenty of fibre, fruit and vegetables and high-fibre carbohydrate foods on the non-diet days.

I'm worried that I won't be able to concentrate at work on my diet days – will I feel less alert?

In our trials a few people – only 3 per cent – found concentration difficult, although it is possible that they were expecting problems and so any effects were exaggerated. There's no consistent evidence that low-calorie or low-carbohydrate diets affect concentration. In one recent study dieters were given either a low-calorie drink or a drink containing their full calorie requirement without being told which drink they were getting. None who received the low-calorie drink reported any problems with concentration, energy levels or mood.[8] Other research suggests that low-carb, high-protein diets could actually increase memory and alertness[9] and have been used to treat older adults with problems with memory and processing information.[10]

If you genuinely feel that you are struggling to concentrate on your diet days make sure you are drinking enough and getting enough sodium, potassium and magnesium, by including recommended foods (see the nutrient list at www. thetwodaydiet.co.uk). Make sure that you are eating enough and getting the permitted amount of carbohydrate allowed on diet days, which you get within your dairy and fruit and vegetable allowances.

'I've been surprised at what you can have for meals and I have never felt hungry if I stick to my drinks and allowed snacks through the day.' Trish, 54

Will my breath smell?

A few dieters complained about a bad taste in their mouth, but this was usually minor and not enough to make their breath smell. The taste is caused by ketones, substances that build up when your body burns fat to use for energy. Although you may notice it on the two diet days, it will disappear on the other five days. Drinking more may help and you can also suck sugar-free mints (up to 10 a day).

Will exercising make me more hungry?

We all react differently to being more active – half of us naturally eat more, the rest eat less or roughly the same amount.[11] As you step up your exercise, monitor your eating and make sure you don't reward yourself or 'compensate' with larger servings or 'treats' of high-sugar, high-fat foods.

Exercise can actually help regulate our appetite and some activity on diet days could help to distract you, especially in the evenings when you might be tempted to break your diet.

'I was a bit worried that exercising on my diet days would make me hungrier and struggle to keep to the diet. Actually going swimming after work gives me a routine, keeps me on track and avoids the evening munchies.' Pat, 54

Troubleshooting

I'm not losing weight – what am I doing wrong?

Make sure that you are sticking to the recommended number of portions on diet and non-diet days and getting enough exercise. You can find Ready Reckoner portion guides for men and women in Appendix A on page 137, which show you how many portions you should be eating based on your age and current weight. Even if you are not seeing an immediate difference on the scales, check to see whether you are losing body fat (see the Body Fat Ready Reckoner on the 2-Day Diet website) and are more toned by taking your waist measurement.

I have to work shifts – how can I make The 2-Day Diet work for me?

Losing weight when you do shift work takes more planning and self-discipline than if you work normal hours. Shift work disrupts your body clock, which can increase your appetite. The good news is that it can be done.

Tips for shift workers:

▶ If you work nights, eat a light meal during the night and a small breakfast after finishing work.

▶ Plan ahead to help you eat as healthily as possible – if necessary take a light meal and healthy snacks to work (see the snack list on page 12).

▶ Drink plenty of water or low-calorie drinks throughout your shift.

▶ Try to get good-quality sleep. Create a good sleep environment and sleep schedule for yourself and stick to it.

▶ Incorporate exercise in your schedule and, if possible, into your breaks at work.

I have diabetes – can I do the diet?

The 2-Day Diet is particularly good for making insulin work more effectively in the body so should help someone with diabetes. However, The 2-Day Diet has not yet been rigorously tested in people with diabetes. The two low-carbohydrate diet days could lead to low blood sugars if you are on insulin or other medicines to control your blood sugars. If you have diabetes seek medical advice before embarking on this or any other diet.

I have tried to lose weight so many times before that I don't know whether it's worth trying again. Has dieting messed up my metabolism?

The 2-Day Diet works not just for first-time dieters but for people who have tried repeatedly to lose weight. Some of our dieters had more than 10 previous attempts! Despite the popular belief, research shows that 'yo-yo' dieters who have tried and failed to lose weight can lose weight just as easily as those who have never been on a diet.[12]

Help – I've broken my diet!

Even dedicated dieters slip up now and again, usually by eating 'forbidden' foods. This is one reason why we have made sure there are treats on The 2-Day Diet! If you do slip, don't beat yourself up or feel like a failure – and certainly don't give up. Just get back on track as soon as you can. If you lapse, try to learn from the experience so you can avoid doing the same thing the next time.

*'It's harder to follow the diet when you are out in
restaurants or at people's houses when they have cooked
for you. You have to make sure you tell them in advance.'*
Diana, 49

Why is my weight loss slowing down?

Weight loss becomes harder when you have been dieting for a
while. Part of this may be due to the inevitable 10–15 per cent
reduction in metabolic rate, which is the body's natural adap-
tation to weight loss and eating less (even when you exercise).

Despite this you should continue to lose weight. Studies
have found that although most weight loss happens in the first
six to eight months of a diet, weight can continue to fall over
three years. So you would lose half of the total weight in the
first year and the second half in the following two years.[13]

Weight loss often slows down because you aren't sticking
as carefully to the diet or exercising as much as when you
first started.

If you feel you are not losing the predicted 0.5–1 kg (1–2
lb) per week, check the following:

▶ Are you following the correct diet plan for someone of
your sex, weight, and age? (See the Ready Reckoners in
Appendix D on page 164.)

▶ Are you overeating on the two diet days?

▶ Are you overeating on the non-diet days or drinking too
much alcohol?

▶ Are you taking the recommended amount of exercise (see
page 24)?

▶ Are you taking every opportunity to be physically active in your daily routine? For example, taking the stairs or aiming to walk rather than drive, where possible?

▶ Keep a tally of your food portions and log your activity diary for four days to check how much you are eating and how active you really are. Remember to include both weekdays and weekends. (Use the tracking tools at www.thetwodaydiet.co.uk)

How can I beat my food cravings?

Most of us have occasional cravings and dieting can make them worse. Some cravings are driven by hunger, but many are triggered by emotional cues. For example, if you feel anxious you might automatically eat biscuits, or you see chocolate at the checkout and pop it in your basket without thinking. Many of our dieters stopped craving sweet things, but sometimes craved bread and other carbs on their diet days. Try to identify your particular triggers and when they happen and reprogramme your brain to overcome these urges.

▶ If you just want to eat something, try having a drink or sugar-free mints.

▶ Distract yourself – phone a friend, have a shower or go for a walk. Although a craving can feel overwhelming, if you can ride it out by diverting yourself it will subside.

▶ Work through the craving, let yourself experience its full force and notice how you think and feel, without giving in to it. It may be hard initially, but learning that you can resist cravings makes it easier next time.[14]

'I do get cravings, but quite often my so-called "hunger" is actually thirst, but even having a few Brazil nuts, cashews, or pecan nuts helps.' Paul, 47

I always get the munchies before my period. What should I do?

A big hurdle for female dieters is managing and overcoming food cravings before your period, especially cravings for high-carbohydrate foods. About half of our dieters struggled with pre-menstrual cravings on their two diet days. These cravings are thought to be the body trying to take in enough carbohydrate to balance levels of chemicals in the brain. If it's too difficult to do your two diet days when you are pre-menstrual, try to reschedule them for when you're not suffering from pre-menstrual munchies.

Sticking to wholegrain carbs on the five non-diet days can help reduce cravings. Calcium, magnesium and vitamin B6 are all thought to help reduce pre-menstrual syndrome and suppress cravings,[15] so eat plenty of foods rich in these nutrients (see www.thetwodaydiet.co.uk).

I suffer from seasonal affective disorder (SAD) in winter. How can I curb my cravings?

Seasonal affective disorder (SAD) is caused by the lack of daylight affecting the chemical balance of the brain and reducing levels of serotonin, a chemical that promotes relaxation and happiness. Whether you have the winter blues or full-blown SAD you will probably notice a craving for starchy and sugary foods, which both help boost levels of serotonin in the brain. So what is the answer? Follow the advice on food cravings, take regular exercise, as it helps to restore the chemical balance of the brain, and try to get as much daylight as possible. Just walking outside for an hour a day has been shown to help SAD sufferers.

Do I need to stick to the diet at Christmas or when I'm on holiday?

Taking a planned diet 'break' shouldn't affect your long-term weight loss. One recent study looked at the impact of a planned two-week diet 'holiday' on people's long-term success. The result? After the break the dieters managed to successfully return to their diets and it did not hamper their long-term success.[16] If you know that you have an event or a special occasion like Christmas or a holiday coming up, plan to deviate from the diet temporarily and then get back on track afterwards.

> *'When I go out for meals I simply have reduced servings to enable me to stick to the diet as I'm never very sure how the food was prepared.' Alicia, 47*

How do I cope with eating out or takeaways?

By being prepared. Restaurant or takeaway meals are usually bigger and higher in calories and fat than meals at home. However, more of them now inform customers about their food's calorie content, so use this information if it is available. Try to avoid fixed-price menus as you may eat more courses and calories than you need or want – because it's included in the price. 'All you can eat' restaurants are also best avoided. Try these tips:

▶ Don't starve yourself before you go out – you could overeat when you eventually have your meal.

▶ Share courses with others or order two starters instead of a starter and main.

▶ Ask how the food is cooked and ask for adaptations (grilling instead of frying for example).

▶ Ask for high-calorie sauces or dressings 'on the side' so you decide how much of them you eat.

▶ Avoid pre-dinner nibbles (crisps, poppadoms) which add lots of extra calories.

▶ Drink plenty of water and less wine.

Am I allowed any alcohol?

You can have an occasional drink, but avoid alcohol completely on diet days and try not to drink more than 10 units a week on non-diet days – this is the equivalent of a bottle of wine, 4½ pints of beer or lager (4%) or 10 pub measures of spirits. Alcohol is packed with calories (a 250 ml glass of wine contains 240 calories and a pint of lager 170 calories) and it makes you less inhibited and more likely to give in to temptation! We know that alcohol consumed before or with meals makes you eat more. Although drinking a little may help protect against heart disease, alcohol can increase the risk of several different cancers including breast, bowel, liver, mouth and oesophageal cancer. Drinks with the fewest calories are spirits with a diet mixer; for example a gin and slimline tonic only contains 50 calories.

Set your maximum limit before you go out for the evening, drink plenty of low-calorie soft drinks or water and avoid salty snacks, which make you thirsty (and are usually full of calories).

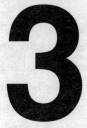

3

Recipes for Diet Days

General note

Most recipes serve one to two people. If you are increasing quantities to feed more people, bear in mind that you may also need to adjust the cooking time. In some cases making a single portion is impractical – soups and stews, especially – and any excess can always be frozen, so that you have a supply of healthy ready meals.

All spoon measurements are level unless otherwise indicated and are assumed to be standard sizes: teaspoon = 5 ml; table-spoon = 15 ml. If you are in any doubt, buy a set of spoon measures. All hobs and ovens differ, so do check as you cook. The oven temperatures given are for conventional electric and gas ovens; for fan-assisted ovens, subtract 20°C from the suggested cooking time.

Salt and sugar

Many of us have developed a preference for salty and sugary foods due to years of eating salty and sweet manufactured foods or habitually adding salt and sugar to flavour our food. Reducing salt and sugar intake is an important component of healthy eating. Cutting down on salt and sugar is quite straightforward: you simply need to get used to eating less. Initially, when you reduce your salt and sugar intake, foods may taste bland or different. You can cut down on salt straight away or reduce your salt intake in 20 per cent steps. Most people can't taste the difference if they reduce salt gradually. Either way, after two or three weeks you will start to taste the genuine, delicious flavours of food. The recipes below include lots of alternative flavourings and do not require salt. Some recipes contain stock and we suggest that you use no more than 2 g/ ¼ stock cube per serving. You can use less than this if you wish or a low-salt bouillon. Try to use tuna, beans and pulses that are tinned in water and not brine or salted water. Similarly, try to use raw prawns, rather than cooked, as these contain much less salt: 100 g (3½ oz) of cooked prawns typically contain 1.1–2 g salt whereas raw prawns contain 0.5 g.

Each recipe shows how many portions it contributes to your allowance in The 2-Day Diet plan. Many foods contain a combination of nutrients, some of which are in such small quantities they do not count towards your portion allowances. All portions have been rounded to the nearest half.

Breakfast

Spicy scrambled eggs
Serves 1

2 eggs
½ tsp rapeseed oil
3 spring onions, chopped
½ mild chilli or to taste,
*   finely chopped (optional)*
¼ tsp turmeric
handful of coriander leaves
1 medium tomato, chopped

PORTIONS		NUTRITIONAL INFO	
Protein	2	Calories	228
Fat	0	Carbohydrate	4 g
Dairy	0	Protein	17 g
Fruit	0	Fibre	2 g
Vegetables	1½	Salt	0.5 g

Beat the eggs in a mug or bowl with a tablespoon of water.

Put the oil in a small non-stick pan over a medium heat. When hot, add the spring onions and chilli (if using) to the pan, and cook gently until the spring onions just begin to colour. Add the turmeric and coriander leaves to the pan and stir for a few seconds, then add the tomato and continue stirring until the tomato is warmed through. Finally, add the beaten egg and cook, stirring constantly, until the egg begins to set. Remove the pan from the heat and serve immediately.

Papaya and golden linseed smoothie

Serves 1

120 g (4 oz) low-fat natural
    yoghurt
juice of ½ a lime
80 g (2¾ oz) ripe papaya,
    skinned and deseeded
5 ice cubes
1 tbp golden linseeds

PORTIONS		NUTRITIONAL INFO	
Protein	0	Calories	112
Fat	½	Carbohydrate	14 g
Dairy	1	Protein	7 g
Fruit	1	Fibre	3 g
Vegetables	0	Salt	0.2 g

Pour the yoghurt and lime juice into a blender and add the
papaya. Blend until smooth (alternatively use a stick blender)
and pour into a large glass over ice. Sprinkle over the linseeds
and serve immediately.

One-dish baked egg, spinach and mushrooms

Serves 1

40 g (1½ oz) chestnut
    mushrooms, sliced
1 clove garlic, peeled and
    crushed
80 g (2¾ oz) baby spinach
    leaves, washed and
    thoroughly dried
½ tsp olive oil
freshly ground black pepper
2 spring onions, sliced

PORTIONS		NUTRITIONAL INFO	
Protein	2	Calories	311
Fat	½	Carbohydrate	3 g
Dairy	1	Protein	29 g
Fruit	0	Fibre	3 g
Vegetables	1½	Salt	1.2 g

2 medium free-range eggs
30 g (1 oz) low-fat Cheddar
    cheese, grated

Preheat the oven to 200°C/400°F/Gas Mark 6. Tip the mushrooms into a mixing bowl and add the garlic, spinach and oil. Season with black pepper and toss until the mushrooms and spinach are coated with garlic and oil.

Spoon the mushrooms and spinach into a small ovenproof dish, then sprinkle over the spring onions. Make two shallow wells and crack an egg into each. Sprinkle over the cheese and bake for 10–15 minutes, until the eggs are just set. Serve immediately.

Tip:

▶ For a peppery hit, replace the spinach with a rocket, spinach and watercress salad.

Soups

Chinese vegetable soup with tofu

Serves 1

250 ml (9 fl oz) low-salt
   vegetable stock
1 small pak choi or half
   a large one, trimmed
   (about 60 g/2 oz)
3 button mushrooms, finely
   sliced
3 spring onions, trimmed
   and finely sliced
1 small piece fresh ginger root
   (about 6 g)

1 garlic clove
150 g (5 oz) firm tofu
dash of light soy sauce

PORTIONS		NUTRITIONAL INFO	
Protein	3	Calories	149
Fat	0	Carbohydrate	6 g
Dairy	0	Protein	15 g
Fruit	0	Fibre	4 g
Vegetables	1½	Salt	1.2 g

Put the stock in a pan and bring it to the boil. Separate the pak choi leaves then slice the stems into thin sticks and the leaves into strips. Put the stems into the stock, together with the mushrooms and the spring onions and lower the heat to a simmer. Grate the ginger and garlic into the pan and cook for 3 minutes.

Cut the tofu into pieces about 1.5 cm (½ in) square. Add the sliced pak choi leaves to the pan and stir them in. Then gently put the tofu in the pan and simmer for a further 2 minutes.

Take the pan off the heat, then using a slotted spoon lift the vegetables and tofu into a serving bowl. Carefully pour the liquid on top and serve immediately with a dash of light soy sauce.

Tip:

▶ Not suitable for freezing.

Cauliflower soup

Serves 1, generously

1 small cauliflower (about 200 g/7 oz)
½ tsp rapeseed oil
½ leek, chopped (about 80 g/ 2¾ oz)
1 garlic clove, crushed
500 ml (17½ fl oz) low-salt vegetable stock
100–150 ml (3½–5 fl oz) semi-skimmed or skimmed milk
black pepper

PORTIONS		NUTRITIONAL INFO	
Protein	0	Calories	182
Fat	0	Carbohydrate	17 g
Dairy	½	Protein	14 g
Fruit	0	Fibre	7 g
Vegetables	3½	Salt	1.1 g

Trim the outer leaves from the cauliflower and split it into florets, cutting away the central stalk – there should be 175 g (6 oz) of cauliflower remaining.

Heat the oil in a pan and add the leek. Stir it for a minute, then add the cauliflower florets and the garlic. Stir these around for a further minute, but don't let them brown; then add the stock. Bring the stock to the boil, reduce the heat and simmer uncovered, until the cauliflower and leek are soft and the liquid is much reduced – about 15 minutes.

Remove the pan from the heat. Blend the soup using a hand blender or place the contents in a liquidiser and blitz, adding enough milk to reach a consistency you like. Return the soup to the pan (if you've used a blender), add black pepper to taste, then reheat and serve.

Tip:

▶ This simple and delicious soup is suitable for making in batches and freezing – just multiply the ingredients as required.

Salads

Zingy smoked salmon salad with avocado
Serves 1

75 g (2½ oz) smoked salmon
black pepper
1 lemon

2 cm (½ in) piece of
cucumber
1 tsp olive oil

½ tsp sesame seeds
small bunch watercress
small bunch rocket leaves
½ small avocado

PORTIONS		NUTRITIONAL INFO	
Protein	2	Calories	226
Fat	2½	Carbohydrate	2 g
Dairy	0	Protein	22 g
Fruit	0	Fibre	3 g
Vegetables	1	Salt	3.6 g

Cut the smoked salmon into strips and put them in a bowl. Grind some black pepper over them and squeeze a little lemon juice over them as well; stir together. Cut the cucumber in half lengthways and remove the seeds, then cut each half in half again lengthways, and finely slice the cucumber sections. Add them to the smoked salmon. Set the bowl aside while you prepare the dressing and assemble the salad.

Put the olive oil in a small bowl and add a squeeze of lemon juice. Whisk or stir them together well and then scatter in the sesame seeds. Tear the leaves from the watercress stalks and put them on a serving plate with the rocket. Peel the avocado and cut it into fine slices. Put these around the salad, then spoon the salmon and cucumber mixture on top. Whisk up the dressing once more and drizzle it over the salad. Serve immediately.

Tip:
▶ As an alternative, make this salad using fresh horseradish instead of the sesame seeds – when it is in season. Grate a little fresh root into the dressing about 30 minutes before assembling the salad. Fresh horseradish can be found at farmers' markets, in good greengrocers or online – and it's best in autumn and winter.

Fish

White fish with tangy watercress sauce
Serves 2

2 cod, haddock or pollack
fillets, approximately
150 g (5 oz) each
2 tsp olive oil

PORTIONS		NUTRITIONAL INFO	
Protein	2½	Calories	184
Fat	½	Carbohydrate	1 g
Dairy	0	Protein	30 g
Fruit	0	Fibre	2 g
Vegetables	1	Salt	0.3 g

For the sauce:
bunch of watercress (about
100 g/3½ oz)   *1 tsp olive oil*
handful of flat-leaf parsley   *large squeeze of lemon juice*
handful of basil leaves   *1 tbsp water*

Make the sauce first. Strip off the watercress leaves, discarding the thickest parts of the stalks and any yellow leaves. Put the leaves in a large jug or liquidiser. Add the parsley and basil leaves, the olive oil and a squeeze of lemon juice. If using a hand blender, pulse the leaves together for a few seconds and then add a little water; if you are using a liquidiser, add some water at the start. Blend until the leaves are thoroughly chopped and there are no large pieces remaining, then pour into a small bowl.

To cook the fish: pat the fillets dry with kitchen paper. Using a non-stick frying pan, heat the olive oil over a medium to low heat. When the oil is hot, add the fish fillets, skin side down. Cook the fillets for 3–5 minutes, depending on how thick they are, then carefully turn over and cook for a little longer until done. The total cooking time should be 5–10 minutes, and the fish is ready when it flakes easily, revealing opaque flesh. Serve immediately, accompanied by some of the sauce (if you have made the sauce in a liquidiser, you may need to drain off some excess liquid first).

Tips:

▶ This dish can be made with any round white fish, and the sauce also goes well with oily fish such as salmon.

▶ On non-diet days you could serve this with new potatoes.

Baked stuffed mackerel
Serves 2

*2 fresh mackerel, gutted and
    heads removed, about
    200 g (7 oz) each
black pepper
several sprigs of thyme
½ a lemon, sliced
1 tbsp lemon juice
½ red onion, sliced (for
    flavour only)*

PORTIONS		NUTRITIONAL INFO	
Protein	7	Calories	270
Fat	0	Carbohydrate	1 g
Dairy	0	Protein	23 g
Fruit	0	Fibre	< 1 g
Vegetables	0	Salt	0.2 g

Preheat the oven to 200°C/400°F/Gas Mark 6. Tear off a large piece of foil and find an ovenproof dish big enough to hold the fish easily.

Place the fish in the middle of the sheet of foil. Season them, both inside and out, with lots of black pepper. Push the thyme into the cavities of the fish, then stuff them further with the slices of lemon and red onion. Bring the foil up around the two fish and add the lemon juice. Then fold the foil over the fish, make a parcel and seal it tightly.

Carefully lift the parcel into the ovenproof dish and put it in the hot oven. Bake the mackerel for 25 minutes then unwrap the parcel carefully, as steam will escape. Remove most of the stuffing, lift the fish on to plates and serve immediately. (If you like, you can quickly remove the skin from the fish and lift off the fillets first.) Serve with a green salad or steamed spinach.

Chicken and turkey

Chicken or turkey stir-fry with mangetout and green beans

Serves 1

1 small chicken breast, about 100 g (3½ oz), skin removed, or turkey breast of the same weight

juice of ½ a lemon

1 tsp light soy sauce

25 g (¾ oz) mangetout, trimmed

50 g (1¾ oz) thin French beans, trimmed

2 spears sprouting broccoli

4 spring onions, sliced diagonally

PORTIONS		NUTRITIONAL INFO	
Protein	3½	Calories	235
Fat	1	Carbohydrate	8 g
Dairy	0	Protein	30 g
Fruit	0	Fibre	6 g
Vegetables	2½	Salt	0.8 g

1 garlic clove, finely chopped

2 cm (½ in) square piece of fresh ginger root, finely chopped

1 small red chilli, deseeded and finely chopped (optional)

2 tsp rapeseed oil

Cut the chicken or turkey breast into strips, no wider than 1 cm (¼ in) and 6 cm (2⅓ in) in length. Put these in a bowl and add a teaspoon of the lemon juice and the soy sauce. Stir to coat, then cover the bowl with clingfilm and put it in the refrigerator for 30 minutes.

Prepare all the vegetables: chop the mangetout and beans into strips the same length as the chicken or turkey pieces; break up the spears of sprouting broccoli and cut off any woody stems; slice the spring onions diagonally and include some of the green part.

Use a non-stick wok or large non-stick frying pan. Put it on a high heat, add the oil and take the chicken or turkey strips out of the refrigerator. Using a slotted spoon, remove the meat from the marinade and put it into the wok – it should spit if the oil is hot enough, so be careful. Cook for about 3–4 minutes, stirring well until it begins to colour, and then remove the meat from the wok and set aside. Add the chopped vegetables, spring onions, garlic, ginger and chilli and cook them quickly until crisp but tender; stir them around or they will stick to the pan and burn. Return the meat and any juices to the wok, add the rest of the lemon juice and allow the chicken to heat up thoroughly, which will take another minute or two. Serve immediately.

Tangy chicken drumsticks with crudités and a harissa dip

Serves 1

2 chicken drumsticks, skin
  removed, about 120 g
  (4 oz) each

For the marinade:
2 spring onions, finely chopped
3 tbsp Worcester sauce
splash Tabasco sauce

black pepper
½ tsp cinnamon
½ tsp ground allspice
¼ tsp ground cumin
3 tsp cider vinegar

PORTIONS		NUTRITIONAL INFO	
Protein	5	Calories	282
Fat	0	Carbohydrate	12 g
Dairy	½	Protein	45 g
Fruit	0	Fibre	3 g
Vegetables	2½	Salt	1 g

For the crudités and dip: 5 cm (2 in) piece of cucumber
3 celery sticks   2 tbsp low-fat Greek yoghurt
3 spring onions   ½ –1 tsp harissa (to taste)

Carefully remove the skin from the drumsticks. Mix all the marinade ingredients together in a small ceramic or glass dish just large enough to hold the two drumsticks. Put the drumsticks in and turn them in the marinade, then spoon some of the marinade over them. Cover with clingfilm and refrigerate for at least 6 hours, but for no longer than 12 hours. Preheat the oven to 190°C/375°F/Gas Mark 5. Lift the chicken out of the marinade, then sieve the remainder of the marinade into a small baking dish (discard the spring onion left in the sieve). Add a tablespoon of water and the chicken drumsticks. Turn them over and over in the marinade and then put the baking dish in the oven. Cook for 35–40 minutes or until the drumsticks are done, which will depend on their size. Turn them over twice during this time.

Prepare the crudités and dip just before the drumsticks are ready. Trim the celery, removing the strings with a knife, and the spring onions. Peel the cucumber, cut it in half, remove the seeds and then slice it into strips. Spoon the yoghurt into a small bowl and gradually add the harissa, tasting it as you go along to make sure that you get the dip just as hot as you want it. Serve with the crudités as soon as the drumsticks are ready.

Tips:

▶ Instead of using individual spices in the marinade, you could use a teaspoon of jerk seasoning; it will taste different, but be equally good. If the brand you choose has a high proportion of chilli in it – they vary – don't use the Tabasco.

▶ The drumsticks can also be served cold.

Vegetarian mains

Ginger, soy and chilli tofu skewers with Chinese leaf and mangetout salad

Serves 1

125 g (4⅓ oz) (half a pack) firm tofu
2 tsp low-salt soy sauce
¼ tsp sesame oil
¼ tsp crushed chilli flakes
2 cm (½ in) piece of root ginger, finely grated

PORTIONS		NUTRITIONAL INFO	
Protein	2½	Calories	151
Fat	0	Carbohydrate	8 g
Dairy	0	Protein	15 g
Fruit	0	Fibre	4 g
Vegetables	2	Salt	1.8 g

For the salad:
⅕ of a head of Chinese leaves, finely sliced
80 g (2¾ oz) mangetout, sliced in half lengthways

½ red chilli, finely chopped
juice of ½ a lime
½ lemongrass stalk, woody outer layers removed and finely sliced

For the skewers, slice the tofu into long strips, approximately 10 cm (4 in) long and 2.5 cm (1 in) wide and thread on to wooden skewers. Transfer the skewers into a baking tray, mix together the soy sauce, sesame oil, chilli flakes and ginger and pour over the skewers. Set aside to marinate for up to an hour, turning the skewers over occasionally to marinate evenly.

Meanwhile, mix together the chilli, lime juice and lemongrass for the dressing.

Preheat the grill to high and grill the skewers for 1–2 minutes each side, until browned.

Toss the salad in the dressing and serve with the skewers and any juices left in the grill pan.

Italian bean stew
Serves 2

1 x 227 g (7½ oz) tin whole
   or chopped plum tomatoes
1 tsp olive oil
1 leek, trimmed and chopped
1 celery stick, chopped
2 garlic cloves, chopped
1 tsp dried mixed herbs,
   Italian if available
160 g (5½ oz) curly kale
   or Savoy cabbage leaves,
   finely chopped

120 g (4 oz) frozen soya
   beans
black pepper

PORTIONS		NUTRITIONAL INFO	
Protein	1	Calories	172
Fat	0	Carbohydrate	11 g
Dairy	0	Protein	14 g
Fruit	0	Fibre	9 g
Vegetables	2½	Salt	0.2 g

Drain the tin of tomatoes over a bowl and set aside the juice. Put a pan over a medium heat and add the oil. Once hot, add the leek and celery and cook them gently, stirring, until they start to soften; don't let them burn. Add the garlic, stir it in and cook for a further minute. Then add the tomatoes, breaking them up as you stir them in, and a sprinkling of the mixed herbs.

Cook very gently for a further 8–10 minutes, stirring regularly, until everything is really tender. Keep an eye on the pan, and if it looks as though the mixture is sticking to the bottom, lower the temperature and add a splash of water. Now add the chopped kale or cabbage and the juice from the tomatoes, and simmer for 15 minutes or so until the kale is thoroughly cooked; again, if it looks as though the liquid may be evaporating too quickly, add a little more water. Finally, add the frozen soya beans and cook the stew for 7–8 minutes, or until the beans are soft but not mushy; adjust the heat if necessary so that you end up with a stew and not a soup (see the tip below). Check the seasoning, add a little black pepper, and serve immediately.

Tips:

▶ This recipe also makes a great thick and chunky soup – just rinse out the tomato tin with water and add that water to the pan to increase the amount of liquid.

▶ Stew or soup, this dish freezes beautifully, and a little grated cheese (such as Edam) is delicious on top.

Mint, feta and soya bean salad
Serves 1

60 g (2 oz) frozen soya beans or fresh edamame
1 tsp olive oil

½ tsp balsamic vinegar
¼ tsp Dijon or wholegrain mustard

2 celery sticks, strings
    removed and finely
    chopped
6 spring onions, chopped
2 cm (½ in) piece of
    cucumber
2 sprigs of fresh mint, leaves
    removed
30 g (1 oz) feta cheese

PORTIONS		NUTRITIONAL INFO	
Protein	1	Calories	220
Fat	½	Carbohydrate	8 g
Dairy	1	Protein	16 g
Fruit	0	Fibre	7 g
Vegetables	2½	Salt	1.4 g

To serve:
handful of lettuce leaves,
    about 60 g (2 oz)
black pepper

Bring a pan of water to the boil and add the frozen soya beans. Return to the boil, then lower the heat and simmer until tender, about 7–8 minutes. Test the beans as they cook and be careful not to overdo them – not only do they go mushy, they also lose their attractive bright-green colour. Cook fresh edamame for a shorter time, until warm and tender. Once cooked, drain and set aside.

Put the oil, vinegar and mustard in a large bowl, beat them together until the mustard is dissolved, and add the warm beans. Stir them well and set the bowl to one side. Prepare the rest of the ingredients: chop the celery and spring onions; partly peel the cucumber along its length, making stripes, then cut in half, remove the seeds and cut the halves across into semi-circles. Take the mint leaves, roll them up and chop them into fine strips. Put all the chopped vegetables and the mint into the bowl with the soya beans, and stir everything together well.

Rinse the feta under running water to get rid of any excess brine.

Put the lettuce leaves on a serving plate, and spoon over the fresh bean salad. Then crumble the feta over the top and add a generous amount of black pepper. Serve immediately.

Roasted vegetables with grilled halloumi
Serves 1

1 slice from a small pumpkin,
   about 80 g (2¾ oz)
½ small aubergine, about
   80 g (2¾ oz) in weight
½ green pepper
1 tsp olive oil
½ large courgette, chopped

PORTIONS		NUTRITIONAL INFO	
Protein	0	Calories	233
Fat	0	Carbohydrate	6 g
Dairy	1½	Protein	15 g
Fruit	0	Fibre	4 g
Vegetables	4	Salt	0.8 g

For the halloumi:
50 g (1¾ oz) low-fat or light
   halloumi, sliced
pinch or two of dried thyme
   or oregano

½ tsp olive oil
handful of fresh oregano
   (optional)

Preheat the oven to 200°C/400°F/Gas Mark 6. Peel the piece of pumpkin and discard any seeds and stringy bits. Cut the firm flesh into chunks of about 1.5 cm (½ in) (you should have about 3 heaped tablespoons). Chop the aubergine and pepper into pieces about the same size. Put the teaspoon of olive oil into a small roasting tin or ovenproof dish and pop it in the oven to warm through. When it is warm, tip the dish so that the oil runs across it, then add the pumpkin, aubergine and pepper. Spread them out, turning each piece in the oil, and put the dish back in the oven for 15 minutes. Then stir the vegetables again and add the chopped courgette. Return the dish to the oven for a further 10 minutes, and check the vegetables for softness – they may take a further 5 minutes or so, depending on the variety of pumpkin used.

When the vegetables are nearly ready, prepare the halloumi. If you have a separate grill and oven, preheat the grill, brush the slices with the oil and rub the herbs into them. Pop the slices on foil and grill both sides.

If your oven and grill are combined, preheat a small nonstick frying pan. Sprinkle both sides of the halloumi slices with a little dried thyme or oregano and add the half-teaspoon of olive oil to the pan. When the pan is hot, fry the halloumi quickly for about a minute on each side.

Put the vegetables on a serving plate, and carefully lift the halloumi beside them. Scatter the fresh oregano over everything, if using, and serve immediately.

Tip:

▶ If you can't find low-fat halloumi you can use low-fat mozzarella instead, but treat it a little differently. Once the roasted vegetables are tender, scatter 50 g (1¾ oz) chopped mozzarella on top; pop the dish under a hot grill until the mozzarella has melted and serve immediately.

Oriental vegetable stir-fry with marinated tofu and cashews

Serves 1

150 g (5 oz) firm tofu
juice of 1 lemon
1 tsp light soy sauce
1 small pak choi or half
*   a large one, trimmed*
*   (about 60 g/2 oz)*

PORTIONS		NUTRITIONAL INFO	
Protein	2½	Calories	286
Fat	1½	Carbohydrate	12 g
Dairy	0	Protein	19 g
Fruit	0	Fibre	6 g
Vegetables	2½	Salt	0.6 g

6 spring onions
1 large garlic clove, finely
  chopped
1–2 cm (¼–½ in) piece of
  fresh ginger root, finely
  chopped

2 tsp rapeseed or other
  neutral-tasting vegetable
  oil
2 handfuls of beansprouts –
  about 4 tbsp
1 tbsp cashew nuts

Carefully cut the block of tofu into slices about 1 cm (¼ in) thick. Put the lemon juice and soy sauce in a dish and blend them together. Spread out a double thickness of kitchen paper, then gently lift the first slice of tofu on to the kitchen paper, fold the paper over and lightly press down on the tofu to blot it. Peel the paper back and then carefully lift the tofu slice into the dish with the marinade. Repeat with the other slices, and then spoon a little of the marinade over the tofu pieces. Cover and leave for 10 minutes, then very carefully turn the slices over. Leave for a further 10 minutes.

Take the pak choi and slice the leaf part into very fine strips then push to one side while you cut the stems into broader pieces. Chop the spring onions diagonally across, including some of the green part. Set these aside with the chopped garlic and ginger.

Heat the oil in a non-stick wok or large non-stick frying pan until it is hot. Get some more kitchen paper, lift the tofu out of the marinade and blot it as before. Cut each slice in half, making rough squares, and gently lower them into the pan. Cook for 3 minutes, and then turn them over carefully. Take the wok off the heat while doing this so the remaining ones don't overcook, then return the wok to the heat and cook the other sides. Have a plate ready, and lift the pieces of tofu on to the plate with a spatula, again doing so with the wok off the heat.

Return the wok to the heat – enough oil should have remained in it – and add the spring onions, the pak choi stems, garlic and ginger. Cook and stir these for 3 minutes, then add the bean sprouts and the pak choi leaf strips. Stir briefly, then add a tablespoon of the marinade and cook it off, stirring. Add the cashew nuts and stir the vegetables around, then carefully replace the tofu. Cook without stirring for a few more seconds, and then transfer the stir-fry to a warm plate. Serve immediately.

Tip:

▶ Tofu can be difficult to handle, but it is worth it; not only is it highly nutritious, but it also takes up flavours beautifully.

Mushroom stew with thyme and feta

Stewed! is a young brand that has given a modern twist to an old-fashioned dish; see their website www.steweduk.co.uk for more information.

Serves 4

45 g (1½ oz) dried porcini mushrooms soaked in 250 ml (9 fl oz) boiling water
50 g (1¾ oz) low-fat, olive-based margarine
16 spring onions, finely sliced
3 garlic cloves, finely sliced
180 g (6 oz) shiitake mushrooms, trimmed and halved

300 g (10 oz) chestnut mushrooms, trimmed and halved

PORTIONS		NUTRITIONAL INFO	
Protein	0	Calories	236
Fat	1½	Carbohydrate	6 g
Dairy	1½	Protein	13 g
Fruit	0	Fibre	4 g
Vegetables	3	Salt	1.9 g

180 g (6 oz) oyster
  mushrooms, torn into
  chunks
4 sprigs fresh thyme
2 bay leaves
250 ml (9 fl oz) low-salt
  vegetable stock

2 tbsp balsamic vinegar
2 tbsp tomato purée
freshly ground black pepper

To serve:
chopped fresh parsley
180 g (6 oz) feta cheese

Begin by soaking the porcini in the boiling water in a bowl for about 20 minutes.

Melt the margarine in a deep, lidded saucepan, add the spring onions and cook on a low heat until softened but not browned.

Add the garlic and cook for a couple more minutes before throwing in your prepared shiitake, chestnut and oyster mushrooms, thyme and bay leaves. The mushrooms will soak up a lot of the fat and juices at first, but don't worry; they will soon let out their own rich juices to moisten the pan again. Cook gently for 10 minutes.

Drain the porcini mushrooms, reserving the soaking liquid, then rinse them under cold water to remove any grit. Once rinsed, add the mushrooms to the cooking stew, give it a good stir and leave to cook gently for 5 more minutes. Line a sieve with some kitchen paper and pour the porcini soaking liquid through to catch any gritty bits. Reserve the strained liquid.

Add the stock, balsamic vinegar and strained porcini soaking liquid, tomato purée and some black pepper. Cover with a lid and cook gently for 20 minutes until the liquid has reduced and you are left with a rich dark stock and tasty mushrooms.

Serve sprinkled with some chopped parsley and crumbled feta cheese.

Tips:

▶ On a non-diet day this stew is delicious served with wholemeal crusty bread or polenta.

▶ As the mushroom stew is very thick it can be also served cold as a salad or as a topping on toasted sourdough.

▶ For non-vegetarians this dish can be served with a lean lamb steak or chicken breast.

▶ You could replace the stock with wine on a non-diet day.

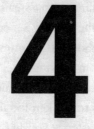

4

Recipes for
Non-diet Days

Breakfast

Porridge with dried fruit
Serves 1

*2 heaped tbsp porridge oats
(about 40 g/1½ oz)*
1 level tsp sultanas
*250 ml (9 fl oz) water or
skimmed or semi-skimmed
milk*
2 dried apricots, chopped

If using skimmed milk:

PORTIONS		NUTRITIONAL INFO	
Carbohydrate	2	Calories	286
Protein	0	Carbohydrate	53 g
Fat	0	Protein	13 g
Dairy	1	Fibre	5 g
Fruit	1	Salt	0.3 g
Vegetables	0		

Put the oats and the sultanas into a small non-stick pan and add the water or milk. Put the pan on a medium heat and bring it to a simmer. Cook for about 10 minutes, stirring frequently to prevent the porridge from sticking.

By now the porridge should be thickening and bubbling well. Stir as it continues to thicken for another few minutes, or until it reaches the consistency you like. Pour into a bowl and scatter the chopped apricots on top. Serve immediately.

Tips:

▶ As an alternative, add 2 chopped almonds to the apricots.

▶ If you prefer your porridge sweeter stir in 1 teaspoon of clear honey.

Classic muesli

Serves 2

80 g (2¾ oz) rolled oats
4 dried apricots, chopped
4 tbsp unsweetened apple
juice
1 dessert apple, unpeeled
2 tbsp low-fat natural
yoghurt
6 Brazil nuts, chopped
2 tsp clear honey (optional)

Without honey:

PORTIONS		NUTRITIONAL INFO	
Carbohydrate	2	Calories	283
Protein	0	Carbohydrate	45 g
Fat	1	Protein	8 g
Dairy	½	Fibre	6 g
Fruit	1	Salt	0.1 g
Vegetables	0		

The evening before you want to eat the muesli, put the oats, chopped apricots and apple juice in a bowl. Stir, cover and leave overnight.

The following morning, grate in the apple and stir well. Add the yoghurt to the mixture and stir that in too. Heat a dry frying pan; when hot, add the chopped nuts, stirring them until they begin to colour. Divide the muesli into two serving bowls and scatter over the toasted nuts. Drizzle the honey over these, if you wish.

Soups

Courgette soup with basil and a tomato salsa
Serves 4

2 tsp olive oil

2 medium onions, peeled and chopped

1 kg (2 lb 4 oz) courgettes, trimmed and roughly chopped

4 garlic cloves, crushed

1 litre (1¾ pints) low-salt vegetable stock

2 medium tomatoes

handful of basil leaves

black pepper

To serve:
4 tbsp low-fat Greek yoghurt

PORTIONS		NUTRITIONAL INFO	
Carbohydrate	0	Calories	146
Protein	0	Carbohydrate	17 g
Fat	0	Protein	9 g
Dairy	½	Fibre	5 g
Fruit	0	Salt	1 g
Vegetables	4		

Put the olive oil in a non-stick pan over a medium heat, and then add the onions. Cook gently, stirring so they don't stick to the bottom of the pan, for about 5 minutes until beginning to soften. Then add the courgettes and garlic and stir these into the softened onions. Cook for a couple of minutes and add the stock, then increase the heat and bring the soup to a simmer. Cook for about 10 minutes, or until the courgettes are soft.

Make the salsa while the soup is cooking. Chop the tomatoes finely and put them in a small dish or bowl. Tear some of the basil leaves and add to the dish with a good twist of black pepper; stir everything together. Set aside while you finish the soup.

When the soup is ready, remove the pan from the heat and allow it to cool a little. Blend it until smooth, using either a hand-held blender or a liquidiser. If you're using a liquidiser, put the soup back into the pan and gently reheat it. Tear up the remaining basil leaves, add them to the pan then pour into the serving bowls. Divide the tomato salsa between the bowls, scattering it in the middle, and add a swirl of Greek yoghurt to each bowl. Serve immediately.

Tips:

▶ If you like bread with your soup, choose a wholemeal variety instead of white.

▶ This recipe is suitable for making in larger batches and freezing. If freezing, don't add the salsa!

Lentil soup with spinach and a touch of lemon
Serves 4

125 g (4⅓ oz) green lentils
250 g (8⅔ oz) fresh spinach leaves
1 tsp olive oil
1 medium onion, chopped
1 garlic clove, finely chopped

PORTIONS		NUTRITIONAL INFO	
Carbohydrate	0	Calories	138
Protein	1½	Carbohydrate	20 g
Fat	0	Protein	10 g
Dairy	0	Fibre	6 g
Fruit	0	Salt	1.1 g
Vegetables	1		

1 tsp tomato purée   *juice of ½ a small lemon*
750–850 ml (1¼ –1½ pints)   *black pepper*
    low-salt vegetable stock

Rinse the lentils in a sieve under running water. Put them in a pan, cover with water and cook over a medium heat for 15–20 minutes, or until they begin to soften. Then drain and rinse them once more. Set aside.

Wash the spinach leaves and remove any really stringy stalks; chop the leaves and tender stalks. Heat the olive oil in a saucepan and add the chopped onion. Cook gently for 10 minutes or until the onion is very soft but not burning, then add the garlic. Cook for a further minute, then stir in the lentils.

Add the wet spinach leaves, plus any chopped stalks to the pan; stir these in. Mix the tomato purée with the stock and add enough of the liquid to the pan to cover the spinach leaves and lentils. Cook for 5 minutes, then add the lemon juice and cook for another 5 minutes (the short cooking time should preserve the vivid green colour of the spinach).

Test that the onions and lentils are really soft and remove the pan from the heat. Allow the soup to cool a little and then blend until it is almost smooth using either a hand-held blender or a liquidiser. If you're using a liquidiser, put the soup back into the pan and gently reheat. Taste for seasoning, adding a little black pepper if you wish, and serve.

Tip:
▶ This recipe is suitable for making into larger batches and freezing.

Roasted tomato soup with pesto

Serves 1

240 g (8½ oz) ripe cherry
   tomatoes
½ tsp chopped thyme leaves
1 stick of celery, roughly
   chopped
2 shallots, peeled and halved
2 cloves of garlic, unpeeled
freshly ground black pepper
1 tsp olive oil
2 tsp balsamic vinegar
1 slice of wholemeal bread,
   cut into bite-sized cubes

250 ml (9 fl oz) hot low-salt
   vegetable stock
1 tsp green pesto
fresh basil leaves, to garnish

PORTIONS		NUTRITIONAL INFO	
Carbohydrate	1	Calories	201
Protein	0	Carbohydrate	26 g
Fat	2	Protein	7 g
Dairy	0	Fibre	6 g
Fruit	0	Salt	1.7 g
Vegetables	3½		

Preheat the oven to 170°C/338°F/Gas Mark 3. Tip the tomatoes, thyme, celery, shallots and garlic into a mixing bowl, season with black pepper and toss with the oil and vinegar. Transfer to a large roasting tin and roast for 45 minutes.

Remove from the oven and stir thoroughly. Scatter the cubes of bread on to a separate baking tray and return both tins to the oven for 15 minutes. After this time the tomatoes, celery and shallots should be golden and semi-dried, and the bread golden and crisp.

Carefully remove the skins from the garlic and spoon the roasted vegetables into a food processor or blender. Add the stock and blend until smooth. Drizzle the pesto over the soup, scatter over the croutons and garnish with basil leaves.

Tip:

▶ This soup is also delicious served cold, like a gazpacho. Serve with a dash of Tabasco to spice it up.

Creamy mushroom soup

Serves 2

2 tsp rapeseed or other
   vegetable oil
2 medium onions, chopped
600 g (1 lb 4 oz) large flat or
   field mushrooms
small pinch cayenne pepper
900 ml (1½ pints) low-salt
   vegetable stock
200 ml (7 fl oz) semi-
   skimmed or skimmed milk
sprig of thyme or a pinch of
   dried mixed herbs
black pepper

To serve:
40 g (1½ oz) no- or low-fat
   Greek yoghurt

PORTIONS		NUTRITIONAL INFO	
Carbohydrate	0	Calories	188
Protein	0	Carbohydrate	20 g
Fat	½	Protein	12 g
Dairy	1	Fibre	6 g
Fruit	0	Salt	1.1 g
Vegetables	5		

Heat the oil in a large pan over a medium heat. Add the onion and cook gently, stirring, for about 5–10 minutes, until soft but not brown. While the onion is cooking, brush any earth from the mushrooms (only peel them if necessary) and trim the ends off the stalks. Chop the mushrooms into chunks. Add the cayenne pepper to the pan and stir for a few seconds before adding the mushroom pieces. Stir these for a further couple of minutes, being careful not to let them burn. Add the stock and milk. Strip the leaves from the thyme sprig into the pan or stir in the dried mixed herbs. Simmer the soup for about 20 minutes, then check for seasoning and add black pepper to taste.

Allow the soup to cool slightly and blend it roughly using either a hand-held blender or a liquidiser – it shouldn't be too smooth. If you are using a liquidiser, add some more water if necessary, then return the soup to the pan and reheat. Serve it with two teaspoons of Greek yoghurt swirled into each bowl.

Tips:

▶ For a chunkier soup, blend only half the soup, and then put it into the pan with the unblended half.

▶ For a more intense flavour use a selection of mushrooms, such as chestnut, forestière or porcini.

▶ This recipe is suitable for making in larger batches and freezing.

Salads

Horiatiki salata – Greek salad
Serves 2

1 small cos lettuce or 2 lettuce
   hearts
4 large ripe tomatoes
½ cucumber, about 180 g
   (6 oz)
1 small red onion or 6 spring
   onions
1 tbsp olive oil

PORTIONS		NUTRITIONAL INFO	
Carbohydrate	0	Calories	265
Protein	0	Carbohydrate	13 g
Fat	2	Protein	11 g
Dairy	1½	Fibre	6 g
Fruit	0	Salt	2.1 g
Vegetables	4		

1 tsp balsamic vinegar   *20 black olives, pitted and sliced*
100 g (3½ oz) feta cheese   *black pepper*

Wash the lettuce leaves, tear them up and divide them between two serving plates or bowls.

Chop the tomatoes and put them in a bowl. Cut the cucumber in half lengthways then chop it up and add to the tomatoes. Then peel the onion, halve it and slice it finely (if using spring onions, chop finely). Add the onion to the bowl. Put the oil and vinegar into a small screw-top jar (a clean jam jar, for instance). Put the lid on securely, then shake to make a dressing. Pour this dressing over the tomatoes, cucumber and onion, and stir everything to combine.

Remove the feta from its packaging and rinse it under running water, then pat dry with kitchen paper. On a plate, cut the feta into small cubes – some brands will crumble and others will require cutting. Slide it into the bowl with the tomatoes. Give this mixture a final, very gentle, stir and spoon it over the salad leaves. Scatter the olives over the salad, add some black pepper and serve.

White bean salad with hard-boiled eggs

Serves 2

2 eggs
½ x 400 g (14 oz) tin haricot
   or cannellini beans
½ x 400 g (14 oz) tin
   blackeyed beans

PORTIONS		NUTRITIONAL INFO	
Carbohydrate	0	Calories	326
Protein	3	Carbohydrate	30 g
Fat	1	Protein	19 g
Dairy	0	Fibre	12 g
Fruit	0	Salt	0.5 g
Vegetables	1½		

1 medium onion, quartered
1 bay leaf
juice of ½ a lemon
1 tbsp olive oil
3 celery sticks, chopped
large handful of flat-leaf
    parsley, chopped

1 small cos lettuce, leaves
    separated
black pepper
10 black olives, pitted and
    halved

Put the eggs in a pan of water and bring to the boil. Cook for 10 minutes, then cool rapidly under a cold tap. Put them in a bowl of iced water and set aside in a cool place.

Drain the tins of beans into a large sieve and rinse them thoroughly. Put the rinsed beans in a large pan over a medium to high heat, add the onion and bay leaf and then cover them with fresh water. Bring the beans to a good rolling simmer and cook for 5 minutes, then drain them well.

Allow the beans to cool a little until they are no longer hot, but still warm; remove the bay leaf and the pieces of onion. Discard the bay leaf, but finely slice two of the onion quarters (or use all if you wish) and put them back into the beans. In a large bowl mix together the lemon juice, olive oil and chopped celery and parsley. Then add the warm beans and onion, and stir everything well. Cover the beans and leave them to absorb the flavours for 30 minutes.

Wash the lettuce leaves, tear them up and divide between two serving plates. Check the flavour of the beans and add black pepper to taste, then stir once more before dividing between the two plates. Peel the hard-boiled eggs and cut these into quarters. Decorate the salad with the eggs and the olives and serve.

Warm beetroot and feta salad
Serves 2

10–12 small to medium
  beetroot, uncooked (about
  150 g/5 oz)
1 bag of mixed salad leaves,
  about 120 g (4 oz)
100 g (3½ oz) feta cheese
1 small red onion, finely
  sliced
1 tsp olive oil
1 tsp lemon juice

leaves from small sprig of
  thyme
black pepper

PORTIONS		NUTRITIONAL INFO	
Carbohydrate	0	Calories	204
Protein	0	Carbohydrate	12 g
Fat	½	Protein	10 g
Dairy	1½	Fibre	4 g
Fruit	0	Salt	2 g
Vegetables	2		

Preheat the oven to 200°C/400°F/Gas Mark 6. Gently clean the raw beetroot but don't scrub, peel or top and tail them; just trim off the leaves, leaving about 1 cm (½ in) of stalk. Tear off a large piece of foil and put the beetroot on it, then seal the foil over to form a flat parcel. Put the parcel on a baking tray and bake in the oven until the beetroot give slightly when you squeeze the parcel; they will take at least 30 minutes, but the cooking time will depend on their size. Test that they are cooked by unwrapping the parcel and sticking a knife in one – it should go in gently, and the skin should also be a little wrinkled.

Carefully unwrap the parcel and allow the beetroot to cool until they can just be handled. Then slide off the skins; these should come away easily, but may need encouragement with a knife. Put the peeled beetroot to one side. (If using cooked beetroot, see tip below; clean them if necessary and pop them in a preheated oven for 5 minutes to warm up – they just need to be warm, not recooked.)

Divide the salad leaves between two plates. Chop the warm beetroot and scatter the pieces over the leaves. Then rinse the feta cheese, pat dry on kitchen paper and crumble it evenly over the beetroot. Scatter the red onion on top, to taste. Make a dressing by whisking together the olive oil, lemon juice and thyme leaves in a small bowl, and pour it over the salad. Add some black pepper and serve immediately.

Tip:

▶ If it is impossible to find raw beetroot, use cooked ones – just omit the roasting instructions; instead, warm briefly as instructed in the method above. If the only raw beetroot you can find are enormous, then definitely use smaller cooked ones.

Tuna and mixed bean salad

Serves 2

1 x 400 g (14 oz) tin of
* mixed beans (pulses) in*
* water*
1 garlic clove, peeled but
* whole*
1 tbsp olive oil
1 tsp balsamic vinegar
½ tsp Dijon mustard
squeeze of lemon juice
10 spring onions, finely sliced

5 radishes, trimmed, halved
* and finely sliced*

PORTIONS		NUTRITIONAL INFO	
Carbohydrate	0	Calories	281
Protein	4	Carbohydrate	25 g
Fat	1	Protein	26 g
Dairy	0	Fibre	11 g
Fruit	0	Salt	0.4 g
Vegetables	1½		

small handful of flat-leaf
   parsley (optional), finely
   chopped
1 x 160–185 g (5½ –6½ oz)
   tin tuna steak in spring
   water

black pepper
1 packet rocket or similarly
   strong-tasting salad
   leaves, about 150 g (5 oz)

Drain and rinse the mixed beans and put them in a pan with the garlic. Cover with fresh water, put the pan over a medium to high heat and bring the beans to a simmer. Turn the heat off and cover the pan; set aside for a couple of minutes while making the dressing.

Put the olive oil, vinegar and mustard in a small bowl and squeeze in some lemon juice. Then whisk well to combine all the ingredients into a vinaigrette dressing. Drain the warm beans, remove the garlic clove, and put the beans in a large bowl. Pour the dressing over them and stir well. Set aside for 10 minutes or so to cool down.

Add the sliced spring onions and radishes to the beans, then the parsley (if using) and stir everything together.

Drain the tuna and flake the fish on to the beans, keeping the flakes as large as possible. Add some black pepper and then carefully mix the tuna and the beans together, trying not to break up the tuna too much. Divide the salad leaves between two plates and spoon the tuna and bean salad on top. Serve immediately.

Tip:
▶ This recipe requires a tin of mixed pulses – generally including chickpeas, borlotti, kidney and haricot beans.

Fish and seafood

Prawns with beans, tomatoes and thyme

Serves 2

*1 x 400 g (14 oz) tin borlotti
    beans*
250 g (8⅔ oz) fresh tomatoes
200 g (7 oz) raw prawns
2 tsp olive oil
1 garlic clove, finely chopped
1 sprig thyme
black pepper

PORTIONS		NUTRITIONAL INFO	
Carbohydrate	0	Calories	241
Protein	4	Carbohydrate	25 g
Fat	½	Protein	27 g
Dairy	0	Fibre	9 g
Fruit	0	Salt	0.6 g
Vegetables	1½		

Drain and rinse the beans. Chop the tomatoes roughly and rinse the prawns under a cold tap.

Put the olive oil in a non-stick frying pan over a medium heat. When it is warm, add the tomatoes and the garlic and cook them together for a couple of minutes. Strip the leaves off the thyme and add them to the pan, and then add the beans. Add the prawns and cook for about 5 minutes until they turn pink and are cooked through. During this time add a little water to keep the mixture from sticking to the bottom of the pan; a couple of tablespoons should be enough – the dish should be lightly sauced – but this will depend on how juicy the tomatoes were. Check for seasoning and add black pepper to taste. Serve immediately, perhaps with wholemeal or crusty granary bread to mop up the sauce.

Tip:

▶ If you cannot buy raw prawns you can use cooked prawns instead, but this will increase the salt content. Cooked prawns should only be gently warmed to avoid overcooking. Add after you have cooked the beans for about 5 minutes.

Salmon with lentils
Serves 2

100 g (3½ oz) Puy lentils
  (uncooked weight)
1 small onion, peeled and
  halved
1 garlic clove, peeled but
  whole
1 bay leaf
1 sprig of thyme
½ tsp olive oil
1 tbsp low-fat cream cheese
black pepper

PORTIONS		NUTRITIONAL INFO	
Carbohydrate	0	Calories	404
Protein	6	Carbohydrate	28 g
Fat	0	Protein	39 g
Dairy	½	Fibre	7 g
Fruit	0	Salt	0.3 g
Vegetables	½		

2 salmon fillets, skin removed,
  approximately 120 g
  (4 oz) each

Rinse the lentils, then put them in a pan with half of the onion, the garlic clove, bay leaf and sprig of thyme. Cover with water and bring to the boil. Reduce the heat to a simmer and cook until the lentils are tender but not soft or mushy. This shouldn't take longer than 30 minutes. Drain the lentils and discard the half onion, garlic, bay leaf and the stalk of the thyme – most of the leaves will have come off.

Finely chop the remaining half onion. Put the oil in a pan over a medium heat and fry the onion gently for 3–4 minutes. Add the lentils and heat through, then take off the heat and allow to cool for 2 or 3 minutes before stirring in the cream cheese. Season with black pepper and cover the pan to keep the lentils warm while you cook the salmon. Heat a non-stick frying pan over a medium to high heat. Place the salmon fillets in the pan and cook them gently on one side for about 2 minutes until they just begin to colour. Then turn them over and cook the other side, also for about 2 minutes. Check the salmon is cooked right through (this will depend on the thickness of the fillets), and take the pan off the heat. Divide the lentils between two warmed plates. Gently place a fillet of salmon on top, and serve immediately.

Tip:

▶ Puy lentils are readily available and don't need preliminary soaking. They also have a lovely nutty taste and are really nutritious.

Chicken

Baked chicken with rosemary

Serves 2

2 skinless chicken breasts,
*   about 125 g (4 oz) each*
1 tsp olive oil
3 sprigs of rosemary
2 garlic cloves, cut into
*   quarters*
juice of 1 lemon

PORTIONS		NUTRITIONAL INFO	
Carbohydrate	0	Calories	159
Protein	4	Carbohydrate	1 g
Fat	0	Protein	28 g
Dairy	0	Fibre	< 1 g
Fruit	0	Salt	0.3 g
Vegetables	0		

Preheat the oven to 200°C/400°F/Gas Mark 6. Remove the skin from the chicken breasts (if not skinless) and discard it.

Drizzle the oil into an ovenproof dish, swirl it around and put the dish in the oven until the oil is hot. Take the dish out of the oven and turn the chicken breasts in the oil to seal them and brown them slightly, then take them out and put them on a plate.

Put the whole sprigs of rosemary in the dish, then scatter in the pieces of garlic. Put the chicken breasts on top of the rosemary, right side up. Make the lemon juice up to 100 ml (3½ fl oz) with water and pour it over the chicken. Return the dish to the oven and cook the chicken for 20 minutes. Then turn the breasts over, cook for a further 5–10 minutes before turning them the right way up again and cooking until they are done: the juice should run clear when you stick a knife into the thickest part. This will probably take another 10 minutes, depending on the size of the chicken breasts. Once the chicken is ready, lift it out of the dish and allow any excess lemony liquid to run off before serving. Serve the breasts immediately, or chill them thoroughly once they have cooled down.

Tips:
▶ These chicken breasts are ideal hot or cold with steamed vegetables, a tomato salad or a baked potato.
▶ Pasta makes a good accompaniment when they're hot, especially if you spoon some of the lemony liquid over the pasta before serving.
▶ Cold and sliced, these are great as a sandwich ingredient or as part of a salad.

Chicken fajitas

Serves 4

500 g (1 lb 1 oz) skinless
    chicken breasts

2 limes

½ tsp paprika

1 tsp ground cumin

1 red chilli, deseeded and
    finely chopped, or ½ tsp
    chilli powder

black pepper

2 tsp olive oil

1 red pepper, deseeded and
    finely chopped

1 green pepper, deseeded and
    finely chopped

1 medium red onion

1 tsp tomato purée

To serve:

salad leaves

bunch of coriander, leaves
    only

150 g (5 oz) low-fat natural
    yoghurt

4 tortilla wraps

PORTIONS		NUTRITIONAL INFO	
Carbohydrate	2	Calories	381
Protein	4	Carbohydrate	49 g
Fat	0	Protein	36 g
Dairy	½	Fibre	5 g
Fruit	0	Salt	0.8 g
Vegetables	2		

Cut the chicken breast into fine strips, no longer than 3.5 cm
(1½ in) and no larger than 1 cm (½ in) deep and wide. Squeeze
one of the limes into a large mixing bowl and add the paprika,
cumin, chilli or chilli powder and a good grinding of black
pepper. Add a teaspoon of olive oil as well, then stir everything
together. Add the chicken and mix it in with a wooden spoon.
Set the bowl to one side.

In the meantime, prepare the peppers, cut the onion in half
and then into slices. Add the vegetables to the chicken bowl,
together with the juice of the other lime, and stir well. Put
some crisp salad leaves on each serving plate, and remove the

leaves from the coriander. Pour the yoghurt into a small bowl. If you want to heat the tortillas in the oven, preheat it and put them in (following the instructions on the packet), or use a microwave.

Warm a large non-stick frying pan or wok on a high heat and add a teaspoon of oil. When smoking, tip in the chicken mixture. Cook, stirring constantly to prevent it burning, for 5 minutes. Then add the tomato purée and stir it in. Continue cooking and stirring for a further minute or until you are sure the chicken is cooked – it should be beginning to crisp a little at the edges and will be opaque all the way through. Remove from the heat. Then assemble the fajitas: spoon some yoghurt on each tortilla wrap, scatter some coriander leaves over it, and divide the chicken between them. Add a little more yoghurt and then wrap the tortilla over. Serve immediately.

Tip:
▷ You can also use turkey breast or steak in this recipe instead of the chicken, and include some guacamole when you wrap the fajitas.

Healthy chicken tagine
Serves 4

2 tsp olive oil

4 free-range skinless chicken breasts, weighing about 120 g (4 oz) each

4 cloves garlic, peeled and crushed

PORTIONS		NUTRITIONAL INFO	
Carbohydrate	2	Calories	368
Protein	4	Carbohydrate	41 g
Fat	½	Protein	34 g
Dairy	0	Fibre	7 g
Fruit	1	Salt	1.2 g
Vegetables	3		

2½ cm (1 in) piece of ginger, peeled and finely grated

2 tsp ground cumin

2 tsp ground coriander

1 tsp ground turmeric

2 small cinnamon sticks

¼ tsp crushed chilli flakes

320 g (11 oz) pumpkin, peeled and cut into bite-sized pieces

500 ml (17 fl oz) hot low-salt chicken stock

4 medium tomatoes, roughly chopped

12 dried apricots, chopped

10 green olives, halved

240 g (8¾ oz) wholemeal couscous

8 spring onions, sliced

1 tbsp each of flat-leaf parsley and mint, torn

240 g (8 oz) green salad, washed and dried

1 lemon, cut into wedges

Begin by heating the oil in a large casserole dish over a medium heat. Add the chicken and fry for 3–4 minutes, turning once, until golden brown. Add the garlic, ginger, cumin, coriander, turmeric, cinnamon sticks and chilli flakes to the pan, and stir to coat the chicken. Cook for 1–2 minutes until fragrant. Tip in the pumpkin pieces and stir to coat in the spice mixture. Pour in the stock, followed by the tomatoes, apricots and olives. Lower the heat, cover and simmer gently for 15–20 minutes, until the chicken has cooked through. Meanwhile, cook the couscous according to the pack instructions. Sprinkle over the spring onions and herbs, divide the tagine between four, and serve with the green salad and lemon wedges.

Tip:

▶ This stew is perfect for freezing. Freeze before adding the herbs and defrost in the fridge overnight before reheating.

Meat

Homemade classic burgers
Serves 4 (makes 4 burgers)

500 g (1 lb 1 oz) lean beef
    mince
black pepper
1 large sprig of thyme, leaves
    stripped
2 tsp Dijon or wholegrain
    mustard (optional)
2 small egg yolks, or 1 large
    one

PORTIONS		NUTRITIONAL INFO	
Carbohydrate	0	Calories	254
Protein	4	Carbohydrate	< 1 g
Fat	0	Protein	29 g
Dairy	0	Fibre	0 g
Fruit	0	Salt	0.6 g
Vegetables	0		

Put the beef in a bowl, grind some black pepper over it and mix it well with a wooden spoon, breaking up any chunks. Then add the leaves from the thyme, the mustard and the egg yolks and combine. The mixture will come together, but do not overwork the meat as it will toughen the burgers. Divide it into four equal amounts and form into four patties. Heat the grill to a high temperature. Put a large piece of foil on the grill pan then carefully lift the patties on to the foil with a spatula. Cook them under the grill for 5–10 minutes, turning once until they are done to your satisfaction. How long this takes will depend on how thick they are as well as how you like them done – rare, medium or well done. Serve immediately.

Vegetarian alternative:
Drain and rinse two 400 g (14 oz) tins of kidney beans in water. Put them in a pan, cover with fresh water and bring to

the boil, then drain the beans again (this makes them easier to mash), and put them in a bowl. Add 100 g (3½ oz) wholemeal breadcrumbs and mash together with the beans, then add the thyme, mustard and egg yolks and stir

SERVINGS		NUTRITIONAL INFO	
Carbohydrate	1	Calories	248
Protein	2	Carbohydrate	41 g
Fat	0	Protein	15 g
Dairy	0	Fibre	10 g
Fruit	0	Salt	0.8 g
Vegetables	0		

everything thoroughly. Form into 4 patties, as above, then put them on a baking tray and grill for 5–6 minutes on each side.

Tips:

▶ These burgers are simple, healthy and quick to make and you can vary the flavourings to suit your personal taste. Try adding some ground cumin, finely chopped chilli and maybe coriander leaves for a hot and spicy burger, or add a bit of cinnamon and cumin for a North African tang.

▶ Baked potatoes and a tomato salad would make a great accompaniment.

Marinated lamb and red onion kebabs with a yoghurt and herb sauce

Serves 2

250 g (8⅔ oz) lean lamb steaks
3 tbsp low-fat natural yoghurt
1 tsp olive oil
1 bay leaf

PORTIONS		NUTRITIONAL INFO	
Carbohydrate	0	Calories	374
Protein	4	Carbohydrate	22 g
Fat	0	Protein	36 g
Dairy	1½	Fibre	2 g
Fruit	0	Salt	0.6 g
Vegetables	½		

black pepper
1 medium red onion

For the sauce:
250 g (8⅔ oz) low- or no-fat
Greek yoghurt

large handful of mint leaves,
finely chopped
pinch paprika

To serve:
handful of coriander leaves

NB: The lamb needs to marinate for several hours or overnight – if it goes into its marinade and into the refrigerator at the start of the day it will be ready to cook that night.

Cut the lamb steaks into 1½ cm (¾ in) cubes, and discard any fat that is easily detached. Put the lamb cubes into a bowl and spoon the 3 tablespoons of yoghurt and oil over them.

Add the bay leaf and turn the meat over in the yoghurt until thoroughly coated. Grind over a little black pepper, cover the bowl with clingfilm and put it in the refrigerator to marinate. If you intend to use bamboo skewers for the kebabs, soak them in water for half an hour before you cook. Make the yoghurt and herb sauce by putting the Greek yoghurt and chopped mint leaves into a bowl. Stir, then sprinkle a little paprika over the top. Pop the dressing in the refrigerator while you prepare and cook the kebabs.

Preheat the grill to a high temperature. Cut the red onion into quarters, then separate each quarter into individual pieces, and take the meat out of the refrigerator. Thread pieces of onion on to the skewers alternately with cubes of meat, then rest the ends of the completed skewers over a roasting tin or baking tray so that the meat is suspended above it. Put the kebabs under the grill and cook, turning them a couple of times until they are done to your taste – this will probably take about 10–15 minutes. Serve immediately with a dollop of the yoghurt sauce and a scatter of coriander leaves.

Chilli and nacho bake

Serves 4

For the chilli:

2 tsp olive oil

1 medium onion, peeled and
    chopped

2 cloves garlic, peeled and
    crushed

1 tsp ground cumin

1–2 tsp chilli powder
    (depending on how hot
    you like it)

480 g (1 lb 1 oz) lean
    minced beef

400 g (14 oz) tin chopped
    tomatoes

400 g (14 oz) tin kidney
    beans, rinsed and drained

250 ml (9 fl oz) hot low-salt
    beef stock

1 tbsp tomato purée

1 large wholemeal tortilla, cut
    into triangles

60 g (2 oz) low-fat Cheddar
    cheese, grated

PORTIONS		NUTRITIONAL INFO	
Carbohydrate	½	Calories	467
Protein	5	Carbohydrate	30 g
Fat	1½	Protein	40 g
Dairy	½	Fibre	9 g
Fruit	0	Salt	1.7 g
Vegetables	2		

4 spring onions, sliced

1–2 tbsp jalepeños, sliced
    (optional)

For the salad:

160 g (5½ oz) romaine or cos
    lettuce leaves, roughly torn

2 medium tomatoes, chopped

1 ripe avocado, stone removed
    and flesh roughly chopped

4 spring onions, sliced

handful of coriander leaves

juice of 1 lime

¼ tsp crushed chilli flakes

Start by making the chilli. Heat half of the oil in a casserole dish
over a medium heat and add the onion. Fry, stirring occasionally
for 5 minutes, until the onion has softened. Add the garlic, cumin
and chilli powder and cook, stirring, for 2 minutes until fragrant.

Remove from the dish with a slotted spoon and transfer to a bowl. Heat the remaining oil and fry the beef mince, breaking it up as you go, until well browned – you may need to do this in two batches. Return the onion and spice mix to the pan and add the chopped tomatoes, kidney beans, stock and tomato purée. Stir thoroughly and bring the mixture to the boil, then lower the heat and simmer, stirring occasionally, for 30 minutes, until the meat is tender and the sauce is nicely reduced.

Preheat the grill to medium/high. Scatter the tortilla triangles over the top of the chilli and scatter over the cheese, spring onions and jalapeños, if using. Place under the grill for 4–5 minutes, until the topping is crisp, golden and melted.

To make the salad, toss together the lettuce, tomatoes and avocado with the spring onions. Sprinkle over the coriander, lime juice and chilli flakes, and divide between four.

Tip:

▶ If your casserole dish won't fit underneath the grill, bake the tortilla-topped chilli in a 200°C/400°F/Gas Mark 6 oven for 8–10 minutes, until the tortillas are crisp at the edges and the cheese melted.

Vegetarian mains

Crunchy stuffed peppers with rocket and raita
Serves 2

75 g (2½ oz) long-grain brown rice

3 large red peppers (or one red, one yellow and one orange)

1½ tsp olive oil

1 large onion, chopped

2 garlic cloves, finely chopped

125 g (4⅓ oz) mushrooms,
   trimmed and sliced

3 tsp pine nuts

10 almonds, roughly chopped

black pepper

100–150 ml (3½ –5 fl oz)
   water

For the salad:

1 bag rocket

1 tsp lemon juice

For the raita:

100 g (3½ oz) low-fat
   natural yoghurt

5 cm (2 in) piece of
   cucumber

PORTIONS		NUTRITIONAL INFO	
Carbohydrate	1½	Calories	431
Protein	0	Carbohydrate	63 g
Fat	2	Protein	15 g
Dairy	½	Fibre	12 g
Fruit	0	Salt	0.2 g
Vegetables	5		

Cook the rice according to the packet instructions.

Preheat the oven to 190°C/375°F/Gas Mark 5. Cut the peppers in half through the stalks, and deseed them without removing the stalk (leaving the stalks on helps the peppers to hold the stuffing). Keeping them intact while removing the seeds is a bit fiddly, but using scissors makes it easier.

Put half a teaspoon of oil on a piece of kitchen paper and wipe the outside of the peppers, then put them in a baking tray, open side up. Bake for 12–15 minutes, depending on their size.

Heat the remaining teaspoon of oil in a non-stick frying pan and add the onion. Cook it for 5 minutes and then add the garlic and the mushrooms. Continue cooking for about 4 minutes, or until the mushrooms and onions are beginning to colour, then add the pine nuts, almonds and a good grinding of black pepper. Stir everything together and take the pan off the heat. Drain the cooked rice, and mix it in with the mushrooms and nuts.

Carefully lift the pepper shells off the baking tray and transfer them to an ovenproof dish (ceramic or glass). Spoon the stuffing into the shells and then pour the water around them – there should be enough to just cover the base of the dish. Put the dish in the oven and bake for 20 minutes.

Prepare the salad and yoghurt sauce while the peppers are cooking. Put the rocket leaves in a serving bowl and toss them together with the lemon juice. Spoon the yoghurt into a small bowl. Grate the cucumber into a sieve; squeeze out as much liquid as possible and then stir the cucumber into the yoghurt. When the peppers are ready, carefully lift them out of whatever water remains in the dish with a large slotted spoon and put them on serving plates. Add a generous spoonful of the yoghurt sauce and serve, accompanied by the lemony rocket. A tomato salsa is another refreshing accompaniment.

Pasta Arrabbiata (and universal tomato sauce)

Serves 2

1 red chilli, or to taste
½ tsp olive oil
1 small onion, chopped
2 garlic cloves, finely chopped
1 x 227 g (8 oz) tin chopped
   tomatoes
150 g (5 oz) dried
   wholewheat penne
basil leaves

For Pasta Arrabbiata:

PORTIONS		NUTRITIONAL INFO	
Carbohydrate	2	Calories	196
Protein	0	Carbohydrate	45 g
Fat	0	Protein	10 g
Dairy	0	Fibre	9 g
Fruit	0	Salt	0.3 g
Vegetables	1½		

For sauce only:

PORTIONS		NUTRITIONAL INFO	
Carbohydrate	0	Calories	48
Protein	0	Carbohydrate	7 g
Fat	0	Protein	2 g
Dairy	0	Fibre	2 g
Fruit	0	Salt	0.1 g
Vegetables	1½		

Be careful when preparing chillies – cut off the top, slice the chilli in half lengthways and scrape out the seeds. Then chop the chilli finely and put it to one side.

To make the tomato sauce, heat the oil in a small pan, add the onions, garlic and chilli. Stir them together and cook very gently for about 10 minutes, or until the onion is transparent and soft. Raise the heat and add the tinned tomatoes. Simmer the sauce until it is reduced by half.

While the sauce is simmering, cook the pasta. Put a large pan of water on to boil. Cook the pasta until it is just ready – about 10 minutes.

You can either serve it as it is or as a smooth tomato sauce. If you want a smooth sauce, put a small sieve over a bowl and pour the sauce into the sieve. Push it through the sieve with a wooden spoon, and scrape the thick sauce into the bowl from the underside of the sieve. Discard the pulp, return the sauce to a clean pan and warm it through.

When the pasta is ready, drain it and put it back in the pan. Add the sauce, either as it comes or smooth, and stir thoroughly to combine. Divide it into two, scatter with a few torn basil leaves and serve.

Universal tomato sauce

For an all-purpose tomato sauce, make the sauce in the same way as described here, but leave out the chilli and include some herbs if you wish – thyme, basil and oregano are particularly good. It should generally be smooth, but that depends on how you wish to use it. It is easy to increase the quantities to make more and any extra sauce can be kept in the refrigerator for two days. It also freezes beautifully.

Tips:

▶ This pasta dish should be spicy hot, but not so hot that it's impossible to eat – and it's lightly sauced.

▶ The basic tomato sauce, without the chilli, can be used in many other recipes.

▶ Serve the pasta with cooked prawns or a sliced roast chicken breast on top.

Bean and green pepper chilli

Serves 4

2 x 400 g (14 oz) tins of
  kidney beans in water
1 x 400 g (14 oz) tin of
  chopped tomatoes
1 large green pepper, deseeded
  and chopped
1 large onion, finely
  chopped
2 garlic cloves, crushed
2 tbsp tomato purée

1 tsp cayenne pepper or chilli
  powder (or more, to taste)

PORTIONS		NUTRITIONAL INFO	
Carbohydrate	2	Calories	390
Protein	2	Carbohydrate	80 g
Fat	0	Protein	17 g
Dairy	0	Fibre	14 g
Fruit	0	Salt	0.2 g
Vegetables	2		

1 tsp ground cumin   ***To serve:***
1 tsp ground coriander   *240 g (8 oz) basmati rice*
black pepper

Drain and rinse the kidney beans and put them in a large pan over a medium heat. Add the tin of tomatoes, and then the chopped pepper and onion. Add the crushed garlic to the pan, followed by the tomato purée, cayenne or chilli powder, ground cumin and coriander. Add some black pepper and stir the pan well, then cover it. Bring it to a steady simmer and cook for 30 minutes. Cook the rice according to packet instructions. Check the chilli as it cooks and give it a stir. If there seems to be a lot of liquid, take the lid off and increase the temperature; if it looks a bit dry, add a little water. The chilli sauce should be thick rather than thin, however. Drain the rice and serve it with the chilli.

Tip:

▶ You could substitute Quorn (300 g/10½ oz) or TVP (textured vegetable protein) (150 g/5 oz) for one of the tins of beans.

Courgette frittata
Serves 2

2 large courgettes (about 150–175 g/5–6 oz total weight), trimmed
2 tsp oil
1 small onion, chopped

PORTIONS		NUTRITIONAL INFO	
Carbohydrate	0	Calories	233
Protein	2	Carbohydrate	4 g
Fat	½	Protein	17 g
Dairy	0	Fibre	2 g
Fruit	0	Salt	0.4 g
Vegetables	1½		

4 eggs
black pepper

Cut the courgettes in half lengthways and then chop them into slices. Warm a teaspoon of the oil in a medium-sized frying pan, add the courgettes and onion and cook over a gentle heat until soft but not floppy. Set the pan to one side.

Beat the eggs in a bowl with some black pepper. Add the courgettes and onion to the eggs, draining off any liquid first if necessary, and mix everything together well.

Wipe the pan with some kitchen paper and put it back on the heat. Add the rest of the oil and allow it to heat, then pour in the courgette and egg mixture. Spread it out, pushing the courgette slices down with a spatula, and tilting the pan so that the liquid egg runs to the edges. Cook gently, shaking the pan slightly to prevent it from sticking, for about 7 minutes or until the underside looks brown when you gently lift it up with the spatula.

Heat the grill, and put the pan under it to cook the top (let the handle stick out). Keep an eye on the frittata, as it will rise and brown quite quickly. Remove the pan from the grill, slide the frittata on to a plate and cut it into quarters. Serve immediately.

Tip:
▶ Potato wedges and steamed green beans make delicious accompaniments.

Aubergine curry with chickpeas, rice and a mango raita
Serves 4

2 medium to large
  aubergines (about
  850 g/1 lb 14 oz total
  weight)
1 x 400 g (14 oz) tin of
  chickpeas
2 cm (½ in) square piece of
  fresh ginger root, peeled
  and finely chopped
2 garlic cloves, finely chopped
1 tbsp rapeseed or other
  neutral-tasting oil
1 large onion, peeled and
  chopped
1 red chilli, finely chopped
  (optional)
2 tsp garam masala
6 tbsp tomato purée

500 ml (17 ½ fl oz) water,
  approximately

To serve:
240 g (8 oz) basmati rice

Mango raita:
300 g (10½ oz) low-fat
  natural yoghurt
2 tsp mango chutney

PORTIONS		NUTRITIONAL INFO	
Carbohydrate	2½	Calories	438
Protein	1	Carbohydrate	81 g
Fat	½	Protein	17 g
Dairy	½	Fibre	14 g
Fruit	0	Salt	0.5 g
Vegetables	3		

Cut the aubergines into slices and then cut the slices into cubes. Drain and rinse the chickpeas and set both to one side. Rinse the rice, put it in a bowl and cover with cold water. Make the raita by putting the yoghurt in a bowl and stirring in the mango chutney. Cover the bowl and put it in the refrigerator. Chop the ginger and the garlic very finely, going over them with a knife until they are almost minced. Heat the oil in a large pan over a medium heat, and add the ginger, garlic paste and chopped onion. Cook, stirring, until the onion is soft but not beginning to colour, then add the chilli (if using) and the garam masala. Cook for a few seconds, still stirring, and then add the aubergine.

Put the tomato purée in a jug and add boiling water; stir, then pour over the aubergine until it is covered. Simmer for 10 minutes. While the aubergine is cooking, put the rice and its soaking water in a pan and cook according to the packet instructions.

When the aubergine has been cooking for 10 minutes, add the chickpeas and cover the pan. Continue cooking for another 10 minutes, keeping an eye on the level of sauce and adding a little water if necessary; give it a good stir to prevent it sticking to the bottom of the pan. If there seems to be a lot of sauce, raise the heat for the last few minutes so that some of it can cook off – this should be quite a dry dish. Serve the curry with the rice as soon as both the rice and the aubergine are ready.

Tips:

▶ The yoghurt sauce (mango raita) that accompanies this curry can also be made by adding a similar quantity of whatever Indian pickle you like, though mango works particularly well with aubergine.

▶ You can also add grated cucumber or onion to the yoghurt for a more authentic raita – squeeze excess moisture out of the cucumber first.

Desserts and baking

Yoghurt ice cream with raspberries

Serves 6

200 g (7 oz) very ripe
raspberries, fresh or frozen
30 g (1 oz) sugar
450 g (15 oz) low-fat
natural yoghurt

PORTIONS		NUTRITIONAL INFO	
Carbohydrate	½	Calories	129
Protein	0	Carbohydrate	19 g
Fat	0	Protein	7 g
Dairy	½	Fibre	3 g
Fruit	½	Salt	0.2 g
Vegetables	0		

Check over the raspberries, removing any small pieces of leaf; rinse them briefly and put them in a bowl. If using frozen berries, defrost before proceeding with the rest of the recipe. Add the sugar and stir it into the raspberries, breaking them up, then add the yoghurt. Blitz everything together using a hand-held blender (or transfer the mixture to a liquidiser). Give the mixture a final stir to make sure it is smooth and that everything is thoroughly blended, then pour it into a shallow freezer container or a similar dish you can safely put in the freezer. Freeze the yoghurt mixture for an hour or until crystals form around the edge. Take it out of the freezer and whisk the mixture thoroughly, then return the container to the freezer. Repeat the whisking after another hour (you can use a hand-held blender – spoon it into a bowl, blend it and return it to the freezer container), and then freeze the ice cream for at least another 2 hours, or until solid.

Take the yoghurt ice cream out of the freezer about 15 minutes before you want to serve it and leave it at room temperature to soften slightly.

Tips:

▶ You can use any berries with this recipe, as long as they are ripe and juicy.

▶ Yoghurt ice cream has a different texture to ice cream made with milk, but whisking it well helps to make it smoother.

Apricot and apple fruit salad

Serves 2

4 dried apricots, chopped
50 ml (1¾ fl oz) apple juice, chilled
4 fresh apricots
2 small dessert apples

PORTIONS		NUTRITIONAL INFO	
Carbohydrate	0	Calories	94
Protein	0	Carbohydrate	23 g
Fat	0	Protein	2 g
Dairy	0	Fibre	5 g
Fruit	2	Salt	< 0.1 g
Vegetables	0		

Put the dried apricots in a bowl. Add the apple juice, cover the bowl and leave it in the refrigerator for at least an hour. Cut up the fresh apricots: halve and remove the stones first, then chop into smaller pieces and add them to the bowl. Cut the apples into fine slices and stir these in. Divide the fruit between two serving bowls and spoon over any apple juice that remains in the larger bowl. Serve immediately.

Tip:

▶ Fresh apricots are delicious, but very seasonal. If you can't find them, choose ripe plums instead.

Baked nectarines stuffed with nuts

Serves 2

2 ripe nectarines
2 level tbsp ground almonds
1 tsp sugar
15 almonds, chopped
1 tsp shelled unsalted
*   pistachios, chopped*
*   (optional, if not using,*
*   add 5 more almonds)*
100 ml (3½ fl oz) orange
*   juice*

PORTIONS		NUTRITIONAL INFO	
Carbohydrate	0	Calories	219
Protein	0	Carbohydrate	18 g
Fat	3	Protein	7 g
Dairy	0	Fibre	4 g
Fruit	1½	Salt	< 0.1 g
Vegetables	0		

Preheat the oven to 200°C/400°F/Gas Mark 6. You will need a small ovenproof dish just big enough to hold four halves of nectarine so that they don't topple over. Halve the nectarines, cutting through to the stone.

Twist one half of each fruit to release it from the stone, and then cut the stone out of the other half. Place the halves in the ovenproof dish, cut side uppermost. Put the ground almonds into a bowl and add the sugar and chopped nuts, then moisten the mixture with a little orange juice until it holds together. Mix well, and then spoon it into the cavities left by the nectarine stones. Pour the rest of the orange juice into the dish around the fruit.

Cover the dish lightly with foil and put it into the oven. Bake for 15 minutes, then remove the foil. Cook for another 5 minutes, or until soft. Gently lift each fruit out of the oven-proof dish with a slotted spoon and put it in a serving bowl. Spoon a little of the juice around each and serve immediately.

Prune delight
Serves 4

200 g (7 oz) pitted prunes
1 tbsp clear honey
250 g (8⅔ oz) low- or no-fat
*   Greek yoghurt*

PORTIONS		NUTRITIONAL INFO	
Carbohydrate	1	Calories	147
Protein	0	Carbohydrate	29 g
Fat	0	Protein	5 g
Dairy	½	Fibre	4 g
Fruit	1½	Salt	0.1 g
Vegetables	0		

Put the prunes into a bowl and pour over a mugful of water; stir, cover and set it aside. Soak them overnight or for several hours.

Empty the prunes and their soaking liquid into a pan over a high heat and bring them to the boil. Then lower the heat and simmer for about 15 minutes, by which time they should be starting to fall apart. Purée them with a hand-held blender or food processor and transfer to a clean bowl; alternatively, push the cooked prunes through a sieve into the bowl with a wooden spoon. Set the prune purée aside and allow it to cool.

Mix the honey and the yoghurt together well, then spoon this mixture into the cooled prunes. Stir together thoroughly and then transfer the mixture into a serving bowl, or into individual ramekins or glasses. Chill for at least an hour before serving.

Tip:
▶ For a fragrant flavour variation, use a scented tea such as Earl Grey as the soaking liquid.

Brown rice pudding with almonds, cinnamon, raisins and orange

Serves 4

120 g (4 oz) short-grain brown rice
375 ml (13 fl oz) semi-skimmed milk
90 g (3 oz) raisins
1 tsp ground cinnamon
4 tsp runny honey
zest of 1 orange, finely grated

PORTIONS		NUTRITIONAL INFO	
Carbohydrate	1½	Calories	239
Protein	0	Carbohydrate	52 g
Fat	0	Protein	6 g
Dairy	½	Fibre	2 g
Fruit	½	Salt	0.2 g
Vegetables	0		

Tip the rice into a medium saucepan and pour over the milk. Cook over a low heat and add the raisins and ground cinnamon. Stir once, cover and simmer very gently for 1 hour, stirring occasionally, until the rice is very tender and the mixture is thick.

Stir in the honey and zest, divide among four bowls and serve immediately.

Tip:

▶ Any dried fruit can be used instead of the raisins. Try using dried cranberries to add a hint of sharpness to the pudding.

Final Word

We've come a long way since we carried out the original research for The 2-Day Diet. Following the publication of the first 2-Day Diet book, we received feedback from many of the thousands of successful Dieters who have lost weight with this approach. If you are trying the diet for the first time – or if you're a veteran 2-Day Dieter, we would love to hear about your experiences and suggestions. You can find us on Facebook (The 2 Day Diet) and join the growing community of Dieters sharing tips, stories and encouragement.

Our research into The 2-Day Diet continues and we are always looking for ways to improve the diet and make it even more effective. We are currently looking at the health benefits of The 2-Day Diet by testing the diet in different groups, including women undergoing treatment for breast cancer. The 2-Day Diet was originally developed as a way for women with breast cancer and those at high risk of the disease to reduce their risk. As with the original 2-Day Diet book and *The 2-Day Diet Cookbook*, all the authors' proceeds from this new book will go directly to Genesis Breast Cancer Prevention, which is the only charity in the UK entirely dedicated to the prevention of breast cancer. You can find out more about our current research by visiting the Genesis website www.genesisuk.org/research.

As well as delivering effective, sustainable weight loss in a way that's easy to build into your life, The 2-Day Diet offers unique health benefits that go beyond shedding unwanted pounds. This new simplified version will make it even easier to reach your goals, get you looking and feeling great and protect your health into the future.

Appendices

Appendix A:
Portion guide for the two diet days

The food lists below show portion sizes for the many different foods allowed on diet days. Try to eat the minimum protein and all of your vegetable, dairy and fruit allowance.

Carbohydrate Foods	Portions
Carbohydrates are not allowed on your two diet days	0

Protein foods

Men and women should aim to have at least four protein portions per diet day. Women can choose up to 12 portions and men up to 14 portions per day. Weights are given for raw meat and fish. Cooked meats will weigh about one-third less than raw, with one portion equivalent to 20 g (¾ oz) cooked meat, poultry and oily fish and 40 g (1½ oz) of cooked white fish. Lean red meat (beef, pork, lamb), bacon and ham are allowed on The-2 Day Diet. However, as they contain some saturated fat, we recommend you limit red meat intake to no more than 700 g (25 oz) raw weight (500 g/18 oz cooked weight) in total per week.

Protein foods	1 portion equal to:
Fresh or smoked white fish (e.g. haddock or cod)	60 g (2 oz) (two fish-finger sized pieces)
Seafood (e.g. prawns, mussels, crab)	45 g (1½ oz)
Tinned tuna in brine or spring water	45 g (1½ oz) drained weight
Oily fish (fresh, smoked or tinned, in tomato sauce or oil, drained) (e.g. mackerel, sardines, salmon, trout, tuna)	30 g (1 oz)
Chicken, turkey, duck, pheasant (cooked without skin)	30 g (1 oz) (a slice the size of a playing card)
Lean beef, pork, lamb, rabbit, venison, offal (fat removed)	30 g (1 oz) (a slice the size of a playing card)
Lean bacon	1 grilled rasher
Lean ham	2 medium or 4 wafer-thin slices
Eggs	1 medium/large egg
Tofu or tempeh	50 g (1¾ oz)

Vegetable protein foods

You can include one of the following vegetable protein foods on each diet day. They count towards your daily protein allowance but do contain some carbohydrate, so try not to exceed the maximum allowance.

Vegetable protein	Maximum per day	Protein portions
Textured vegetable protein (TVP)	30 g (1 oz)	3
Soya and edamame beans	60 g (2 oz)	2
Low-fat hummus	1 heaped tablespoon	1
Quorn	115 g (4 oz)	4
Vegetarian sausage	1 sausage	2
Roast soya beans	15 g (½ oz)	1

Fat

Women can choose up to five and men up to six portions from the list below per day. Note that nuts and avocados count towards your fat allowance, not your protein or fruit and vegetable allowances.

Fats and high-fat foods	1 portion equal to:
Margarine or low-fat spread (avoid the 'buttery' types)	1 teaspoon (8 g)
Olive oil or other oil (not palm, coconut or ghee)	1 dessertspoon (7 g)
Oil-based dressing	1 dessertspoon (7 g)
Any unsalted or salted or dry-roasted nuts except chestnuts (not honey roast), seeds (e.g. sesame or linseed)	1 dessertspoon (8 g) (not chestnuts)
Pesto	1 teaspoon (8 g)
Mayonnaise	1 teaspoon (5 g)
Low-fat mayonnaise	1 tablespoon (15 g)
Olives	10
Peanut or other nut butter (without palm oil)	1 teaspoon (8 g)
Cocoa powder	2 heaped teaspoons (12 g)

Other high-fat foods

You can only have one of the following fatty foods on each diet day as they contain some carbohydrate. They count towards your daily fat allowance.

Fat	Maximum per day	Number of fat portions
Avocado	½	2
Guacamole	2 tablespoons	2
Low-fat guacamole	2 tablespoons	1

Low-fat dairy foods

You should aim to have three dairy portions per day. Mix and match from the list below within your daily allowance. Don't forget that the milk you have in tea and coffee is part of your daily dairy allowance. Lower-fat cheeses are allowed on The 2-Day Diet. These cheeses contain some saturated fat so we recommend limiting them to no more than 150 g (5 oz) per week in total.

Dairy	1 portion equal to:
Milk (semi-skimmed or skimmed)	200 ml (⅓ pint/7 fl oz)
Soya milk (sweetened or unsweetened with added calcium)	200 ml (⅓ pint/7 fl oz)
Yoghurt: diet fruit, plain soya; Greek, plain or fromage frais (all low fat)	1 small pot 120–150 g (4–5 oz) or 3 heaped tablespoons
Whole milk plain yoghurt	80–90 g (2½–3 oz) or 2 heaped tablespoons
Cottage cheese	75 g (2½ oz) or 2 tablespoons
Quark	⅓ pot or 3 tablespoons (90 g/3 oz)
Cream cheese (light or extra-light)	1 tablespoon (30 g/1 oz)
Lower-fat cheeses: reduced-fat Cheddar, Edam, Bavarian smoked, feta, Camembert, ricotta, mozzarella, reduced-fat halloumi, paneer made from semi-skimmed milk	30 g (1 oz)

The dairy-free 2-Day Diet

If you don't eat dairy foods you can replace your dairy portions with the equivalent quantities of calcium-fortified soya milk, yoghurts or unsweetened nut milks. You can also use rice or oat milk on your non-diet days, but not on diet days as they are too high in carbs.

If you don't want to use one of these milk alternatives, you can replace milk with 6 vegetable protein portions (see vegetable protein table on page 138). These vegetable protein portions are in addition to your standard protein allowance (4–12 portions for women and 4–14 portions for men). Make sure you include plenty of non-dairy calcium in your diet from almonds, eggs, beans and leafy green vegetables, tinned oily fish (if you eat the bones) and tofu with added calcium.

Vegetables

Choose five portions of vegetables from the list below per day. Vegetables can be raw, cooked or pickled. Only low-carbohydrate vegetables are allowed on the diet days. Higher-carbohydrate vegetables, such as carrots, other root vegetables and onions are not included on diet days but are encouraged on the non-diet days.

Vegetable	1 portion equal to 80 g (2½ oz) or:
Artichoke	2 globe hearts
Asparagus, tinned	7 spears
Asparagus, fresh	5 spears

The 2-Day Diet: The Quick & Easy Edition

Vegetable	1 portion equal to 80 g (2½ oz) or:
Aubergine	⅓ medium
Beans, French	4 heaped tablespoons
Beans, runner	4 heaped tablespoons
Beansprouts, fresh	2 handfuls
Broccoli	2 florets
Brussels sprouts	8
Cabbage	⅛ small cabbage or 3 heaped tablespoons of shredded cabbage
Cauliflower	8 florets
Celeriac	3 heaped tablespoons
Celery	3 sticks
Chinese leaves	⅕ head
Courgette	½ large
Cucumber	5 cm (2 in) piece
Curly kale, cooked	4 heaped tablespoons
Fennel	½ cup sliced
Kerela or gourd	½
Leeks	1 medium
Lettuce (mixed leaves or rocket)	1 cereal bowlful
Mangetout	1 handful
Mushrooms, fresh	14 button or 3 handfuls of sliced
Mushrooms, dried	2 tablespoons or handful porcini
Okra	16 medium
Pak choi (Chinese cabbage)	2 handfuls
Pepper (green only)	½

Vegetable	1 portion equal to 80 g (2½ oz) or:
Pumpkin	3 heaped tablespoons
Radish	10
Spinach, cooked	2 heaped tablespoons
Spinach, fresh	1 cereal bowlful
Spring greens, cooked	4 heaped tablespoons
Spring onion	8
Sweetcorn, baby (whole not kernels)	6
Tomato, tinned	2 plum tomatoes or ½ tin chopped
Tomato, fresh	1 medium or 7 cherry
Tomato, purée	1 heaped tablespoon
Tomato, sundried	4 pieces
Watercress	1 cereal bowlful

Fruit

You can have 1 portion (80 g/2½ oz) of fruit on each of your diet days. Avoid high-carbohydrate fruits such as bananas, blueberries, grapes, mango, pomegranate, Sharon fruit, fruit juice or tinned fruit, fresh or dried figs and dates and all other dried fruit (except for dried apricots). These high-carbohydrate fruits are encouraged on your non-diet days.

Fruit	1 portion equal to 80 g (2½ oz) or:
Berries (e.g. blackberries, redcurrants, raspberries, strawberries)	1 handful
Cherries	15
Dried apricots	3

Fruit	1 portion equal to 80 g (2½ oz) or:
Grapefruit, guava	½ whole fruit
Large fruit (e.g. melon, pineapple, papaya)	1 slice
Medium fruit (e.g. apple, kiwi, nectarine, orange, peach, pear)	1
Small fruits (e.g. fresh apricots, clementines, passion fruit, plums)	2
Any stewed fruit – unsweetened or with sweetener (e.g. apple, rhubarb)	3 tablespoons
Kumquats, lychees, physalis	5

Flavourings

You can use the following flavourings freely on diet days: lemon juice; fresh or dried herbs; spices; black pepper; mustard; horse-radish; vinegars; garlic; fresh or pre-chopped; chilli, fresh or dried; soy sauce; miso paste; fish sauce; Worcester sauce.

Drinks

Aim to drink at least eight drinks or 2 litres (4 pints) per day on your diet days.

Drinks	Recommended amount
Water (still or sparkling)	Unlimited
Tea and coffee, caffeinated or decaffeinated	Unlimited
Fruit, herbal or green teas	Unlimited
Sugar-free or diet squash or fizzy drinks	Up to 3 litres (6 pints) or up to a maximum of 9 cans per week in total

The Vegetarian 2-Day Diet

We have adapted The 2-Day Diet for vegetarians. Some vegetarian sources of protein contain carbohydrates. Milk and yoghurt also contain some carbs so we have slightly reduced the amounts of these on diet days to keep the carbs down. Your selection of protein foods is more limited than for meat- and fish-eaters, but make sure you include the recommended amounts of protein and low-fat dairy foods so that you don't get hungry. Vegetarians can eat the same amount of fat, vegetables and fruit as those not following the standard 2-Day Diet (see page 137).

Carbohydrate foods

Carbohydrate Foods	Portions
Carbohydrates are not allowed on your two diet days	0

Protein foods

Men and women should aim to have at least four protein portions per day. Women can choose up to 12 portions and men up to 14 portions per day. On your two diet days of The 2-Day Diet you can have generous amounts of eggs and tofu within your daily allowance:

Protein foods	1 portion equal to:
Egg	1 medium/large egg
Tofu and tempeh	50 g (1¾ oz)

You can also choose up to six vegetarian protein portions from the following list each day:

Vegetable protein	Maximum per day	Number protein portions
Textured vegetable protein (TVP)	30 g (1 oz)	3
Soya and edamame beans	60 g (2 oz)	2
Low-fat hummus	1 heaped tablespoon	1
Quorn	115 g (4 oz)	4
Vegetarian sausage	1 sausage	2
Roast soya beans	15 g (½ oz)	1

Dairy foods

You can have up to 60 g (2 oz) of lower-fat cheese, on each diet day (e.g. reduced-fat Cheddar, feta, mozzarella, Bavarian smoked cheese, Camembert, Edam, ricotta, reduced-fat halloumi).

You can also choose two dairy portions from the following list per diet day. Don't use rice or oat milk instead of dairy or soya milk. They are unsuitable for diet days as they are too high in carbohydrates. You can use them on non-diet days.

Dairy	1 portion equal to:
Milk (semi-skimmed or skimmed)	200 ml (⅓ pint/7 fl oz)
Soya milk (sweetened or unsweetened with added calcium)	200 ml (⅓ pint/7 fl oz)
Yoghurt: diet fruit, plain soya; Greek, plain or fromage frais (all low fat)	1 small pot 120–150 g (4–5 oz) or 3 heaped tablespoons
Whole milk plain yoghurt	80–90 g (2½–3 oz) or 2 heaped tablespoons
Cottage cheese	75 g (2½ oz) or 2 tablespoons
Quark	⅓ pot/3 tablespoons (90 g/3 oz)
Cream cheese (light or extra-light)	1 tablespoon (30 g/1 oz)

Appendix B:
Portion guide for non-diet days

We encourage you to follow a healthy Mediterranean diet on your non-diet days. The Mediterranean diet allows you a wider range of foods than your two diet days and includes carbohydrates, protein, low-fat dairy foods and a wide variety of fruits and vegetables. The tables below are a guide to what makes up a single portion of a given food. You should tailor the amount you eat from each food group depending on your gender, weight and age. The tables in Appendix D outline the right quantity of these portions for you. Foods marked with an asterisk are high in salt. Try to limit these salty foods to once during your five non-diet days.

Carbohydrate foods

Recommended amounts vary – check the Ready Reckoner in Appendix D.

Carbohydrate foods	1 portion equal to:
Wholewheat or oat breakfast cereal	3 level tablespoons (24 g/¾ oz)
Wholewheat or oat bisk	1 bisk
Porridge oats or sugar-free muesli	1 heaped tablespoon (20 g/⅔ oz)
Wholegrain, wholemeal, rye, granary bread	1 medium slice, ½ roll
Pitta bread, chapatti, tortilla wrap (wholemeal or multigrain versions)	½ large
Rye crispbread	2
Wholewheat cracker	2

Carbohydrate foods	1 portion equal to:
Oat cake (choose a variety without palm oil)	1
Dried wholegrain pasta or rice	1 tablespoon uncooked (30 g/ 1 oz) or 2 tablespoons cooked (60 g/2 oz)
Couscous, bulgur wheat, pearl barley, quinoa	1 tablespoon uncooked (30 g/ 1 oz) or 2 tablespoons cooked (60 g/2 oz)
Lasagne (preferably wholemeal)	1 sheet
Noodles (preferably brown)	Half a dried block or nest (50 g/ 1oz)
Baked or boiled potato (in skin)	1 small (120 g/4 oz) raw weight
Cassava, yam, sweet potato	1 small (90 g/3 oz) raw weight
Wholemeal pizza base	⅙ of thin medium pizza base
Sweetcorn	½ corn on the cob or 2 tablespoons kernels
Wholemeal flour	1 level tablespoon
Unsweetened popcorn	20 g (⅔ oz)

Protein foods

Recommended amounts vary – check the Ready Reckoner in Appendix D. For optimum health we recommend that you limit red meat intake to no more than 700 g (25 oz) raw weight, 500 g (18 oz) cooked weight per week in total.

Protein foods	1 portion equal to:
Fresh or smoked* white fish (for example, haddock or cod)	60 g (2 oz) (two fish finger-sized pieces)
Tinned tuna in brine or spring water (drained weight)	45 g (1½ oz)
Oily fish (fresh, smoked or tinned, in tomato sauce or oil, drained), (e.g. mackerel, salmon, trout, tuna)	30 g (1 oz)
Seafood, e.g. prawns, mussels, crab	45 g (1½ oz)
Chicken, turkey or duck (cooked without the skin)	30 g (1 oz) (a slice the size of a playing card)
Lean beef, pork, lamb, rabbit, venison or offal (fat removed)	30 g (1 oz)
Lean bacon*	1 rasher
Lean ham*	2 medium or 4 wafer-thin slices
Eggs	1 medium/large

Vegetable protein	1 portion equal to:
Baked beans	2 level tablespoons (60 g/2 oz)
Lentils, chickpeas and beans	1 tablespoon (20 g/ ⅔ oz) raw or 1½ tablespoons cooked or tinned (65 g/2 oz)
Quorn, e.g. pieces, mince, fillets	30 g (1 oz)
Vegetarian sausage	½
Tofu or tempeh	⅛ of packet (50 g/1¾ oz)
Textured vegetable protein (TVP)	1 heaped tablespoon (10 g/⅓ oz) uncooked
Frozen vegetarian mince	30 g (1 oz)
Low-fat hummus	1 heaped tablespoon (30 g/1 oz)
Soya and edamame beans	30 g (1 oz)
Roast soya beans	15 g (½ oz)

Fat

Recommended amounts vary – check the Ready Reckoner in Appendix D.

Fats and high-fat foods	1 portion equal to:
Margarine or low-fat spread, avoid the buttery types	1 teaspoon (8 g)
Olive oil or other oil	1 dessertspoon (7 g)
Oil-based dressing	1 dessertspoon (7 g)
Unsalted nuts/seeds (e.g. sesame, linseed)	1 dessertspoon or 3 walnut halves, 3 Brazil nuts, 4 almonds, 8 peanuts, 10 cashews or pistachios
Avocado	¼ average pear
Pesto	1 level teaspoon (8 g)
Olives*	10
Mayonnaise	1 teaspoon (5 g)
Low-fat mayonnaise	1 tablespoon (15 g)
Guacamole	1 tablespoon (15 g)
Low-fat guacamole	2 tablespoons (30 g)
Peanut butter (choose a variety without palm oil)	1 heaped teaspoon (11 g)
Curry paste	1 level tablespoon (15 g)
Cocoa powder	2 heaped teaspoons (12 g)

Milk and low-fat dairy foods

You should aim to have three dairy portions per day from the list below. Don't forget that the milk you have in tea and coffee is part of your daily dairy allowance. Lower-fat cheeses like Edam or low-fat Cheddar or Camembert are allowed. These still contain some saturated fat so we recommend limiting these to no more than 150 g (5 oz) per week in total.

Dairy foods	1 portion equal to:
Milk (semi-skimmed or skimmed)	200 ml (⅓ pint/7 fl oz)
Alternative 'milks', e.g. soya, oat (sweetened or unsweetened)	200 ml (⅓ pint/7 fl oz)
Reduced-fat evaporated milk	1 level tablespoon (15 g)
Yoghurt: diet fruit, plain soya; Greek, plain or fromage frais (all low-fat)	1 small pot (120–150 g/4–5 oz) or 3 heaped tablespoons
Yoghurt: low-fat fruit, whole milk fruit and plain, flavoured soya yoghurt	80–90 g (2½–3 oz) or 2 heaped tablespoons
Cottage cheese	¼ pot (75 g/2½ oz) or 2 tablespoons
Cream cheese (light or extra-light)	1 level tablespoon (30 g/1 oz)
Quark	⅓ pot or 3 level tablespoons (90 g/ 3 oz)
Lower-fat cheeses: reduced-fat Cheddar, Edam, Bavarian smoked, feta,* Camembert, ricotta, mozzarella, reduced-fat halloumi, paneer made from semi-skimmed milk	Matchbox-sized 30 g (1 oz)

*Try to limit these salty foods to once during your five non-diet days

Vegetables

Choose at least five portions a day of any vegetables you like (except potato, yam, sweetcorn, which are counted as carbohydrate). We recommend you only have one glass of vegetable juice per day as it is better to eat vegetables, which are a great source of fibre.

Vegetables	1 portion equal to 80 g (2½ oz) or:
Any boiled or steamed vegetables	2–3 heaped tablespoons
Salad	1 bowl
Homemade vegetable soup	½ bowl
Vegetable juice	200 ml (⅓ pint/7 fl oz)
Tomato purée	1 level tablespoon

Fruit

You can include any type of fruit on your non-diet days. We recommend two portions per day. Try to limit yourself to one glass of fruit juice per day as it is better to eat whole fruit, which is an important source of fibre.

Fruit	1 portion equal to 80 g (2½ oz) or:
Banana	1 small
Berries (e.g. blueberries, blackberries, redcurrants, raspberries, strawberries)	1 handful
Dried fruit	3 dried apricots; 3 small figs; 3 small dates; 1 handful of raisins
Fruit juice	1 small glass (125 ml/4 fl oz)
Grapes, cherries	15
Grapefruit, guava	½ whole fruit
Large fruit (e.g. mango, melon, pineapple, papaya)	1 slice
Medium fruit (e.g. apple, kiwi, nectarine, orange, peach, pear, pomegranate, Sharon fruit)	1 fruit
Small fruit (e.g. apricots, clementines, fresh dates, fresh figs, passion fruit, plums)	2 fruits

Fruit	1 portion equal to 80 g (2½ oz) or:
Any stewed fruit, unsweetened or with sweetener (e.g. apple, cranberry, rhubarb)	3 level tablespoons
Any tinned fruit in natural juice	3 level tablespoons
Prepacked fruit salads	80 g (2½ oz)
Kumquats, lychees, physalis	5 fruits

Drinks

Aim to drink at least eight drinks or 2 litres (4 pints) a day on your diet days.

Drinks	Recommended amount
Water (still or sparkling)	Unlimited
Tea and coffee, caffeinated or decaffeinated	Unlimited
Fruit, herbal or green teas	Unlimited
Sugar-free or diet squash or fizzy drinks	Up to 3 litres (6 pints) or up to a maximum of 9 cans per week, i.e diet and non-diet days

Alcohol

Alcohol (up to a maximum of 10 units alcohol per week)	Units of alcohol	Calories
Wine 13% (250 ml/9 fl oz)	3.3	240
Cider (568 ml/1 pint bottle)	2.3	210
Pint of beer/lager 4% (568 ml/1 pint)	2.3	170
Wine 13% (175 ml/6 fl oz)	2.3	170

Champagne (125 ml/4 fl oz)	1.5	100
Alcopop 5% (275 ml/9 fl oz bottle)	1.4	200
Port (50 ml/1¾ fl oz)	1	79
Sherry (50 ml/1¾ fl oz)	1	58
Gin (25 ml/1 fl oz) and slimline tonic	1	50

Treats

You can include up to three treat foods a week on your non-diet days. Examples of possible treats you may want to include are:

Treats	1 portion equal to:
Crisps	1 small packet (25–30 g/¾–1 oz)
Plain or chocolate biscuits (e.g. digestive)	2
Chocolate (ideally dark 70% cocoa or higher content)	5 small squares or 30 g (1 oz)
Malt loaf	1 slice
Hot cross bun	1 bun
Fruity teacake	1 teacake
Fairy cakes	2 small cakes with thin or no icing
Flapjack	2 'mini bites' (3 cm/1 in square)
Jaffa cakes, ginger nuts or small chocolate chip cookies	3
Individual chocolate or truffle	3
Rich Tea biscuits	4
Chocolate bar	½ a 58 g bar or a funsize bar
Cereal bar	1
Honey or jam	1–2 tablespoons

Appendix C:
Two weeks of sample meal plans

Here are some suggested meal plans to help guide you through the early weeks of The 2-Day Diet – until the 2-Day pattern of eating becomes established. We've given you two weeks of menu suggestions, with your diet days falling on a Monday and Tuesday, which are popular diet days for many 2-Day Dieters. You can, of course, swap them around if other days work better for you. It is a good idea to stick to the same two days each week, so that The 2-Day Diet becomes a habit. Some people find it better to diet on days when they are busy, whereas others find it preferable to diet on quieter days.

This section includes both standard and vegetarian plans that combine easy-to-prepare recipes with quick, healthy meals. Use the meal planners in whatever way works best for you. Some Dieters find that sticking closely to suggested meal plans helps them to stay focused, especially at the beginning of The 2-Day Diet. For those who want a little more flexibility, the meal plans will provide a great starting point to mix and match meal ideas.

Two dairy portions have been included in each day and it is assumed that one additional dairy portion will be used in the form of milk in drinks such as tea and coffee throughout the day.

The amounts of food in the meal plans are suitable for a woman who is aged 30–60 years and weighs between 10½ and 11½ stone. You will need to adjust the amounts depending on your gender, age and weight. Check the Ready Reckoners (pages 164–171) and food quantity lists (pages 137–154) to determine the appropriate portion size for you.

The 2-Day Diet: The Quick & Easy Edition

Week 1 Monday–Thursday

	Monday	Tuesday	Wednesday	Thursday
Breakfast	2 rashers grilled bacon ½ tin plum tomatoes Milky coffee (200 ml milk)	Recipe: One-dish baked egg, spinach and mushrooms	Recipe: Porridge with dried fruit	2 slices granary toast with 2 tsp low-fat spread and 1 scrambled egg
Mid-morning snack	1 tbsp cottage cheese		20 g unsweetened popcorn	1 apricot
Lunch	Recipe: Cauliflower soup	Vegetable crudités with 1 tbsp each of low-fat hummus and low-fat cream cheese	Recipe: Tuna and mixed bean salad with: 3 crispbreads	Recipe: Warm beetroot and feta salad, served with 240 g new potatoes
			A small pot of yoghurt	
Mid-afternoon snack	Slice of melon		Apple	
Evening meal	Recipe: Baked stuffed mackerel served with a large serving of steamed broccoli	Recipe: Chicken or turkey stir-fry with mangetout and green beans	Recipe: Baked chicken with rosemary, served with: 4 tbsp bulgar wheat and 3 servings of steamed vegetables	Recipe: Chilli and nacho bake served with large mixed salad
		7 strawberries		Recipe: Prune delight
Supper	Handful of almonds and 10 olives	2 celery sticks and 2 tsp peanut butter	Handful of walnuts	1 oatcake and 1 tbsp low-fat hummus
Drinks	200 ml milk in drinks throughout the day	200 ml milk in drinks throughout the day	200 ml milk in drinks throughout the day	200ml milk in drinks throughout the day

Week 1 Friday–Sunday

	Friday	Saturday	Sunday
Breakfast	3 tbsp bran-based cereal with 200 ml milk	2 slices of wholemeal toast, 2 tsps olive spread and low-sugar jam	Recipe: Classic muesli
Mid-morning snack	1 satsuma	1 tbsp low-fat hummus with pepper and carrot sticks	Handful of Brazil nuts
Lunch	Recipe: Lentil soup with spinach and a touch of lemon, served with a chicken salad sandwich on 2 slices of wholemeal bread with 1 tbsp low-fat mayonnaise	4 wholewheat crackers with 1tbsp low-fat cream cheese plus 1 bowl mixed salad with: 60 g salmon, 1 tbsp butter beans, with 2 tsp olive oil dressing	2 slices rye toast with 2 tsp low-fat spread and 4 tbsp baked beans 7 cherry tomatoes
Mid-afternoon snack	30 g low-fat Cheddar cheese and 3 rye crispbreads	Apple and 1 satsuma	200 ml glass of vegetable juice 2 oat cakes and 1tbsp low fat cream cheese
Evening meal	120 g grilled sardines served with: 240 g new potatoes and 4–6 tbsp steamed vegetables Recipe: Baked nectarines stuffed with nuts	Recipe: Chicken fajitas, served with large mixed salad Recipe: Yoghurt ice cream with raspberries	Recipe: Salmon with lentils 6–8 tbsp steamed green veg
Supper	Vegetable crudités and tomato salsa		2 clementines
Drinks	200 ml milk in drinks throughout the day	200 ml milk in drinks throughout the day	200 ml milk in drinks throughout the day

Week 2 Monday–Thursday

Meal	Monday	Tuesday	Wednesday	Thursday
Breakfast	Half a grapefruit Recipe: Spicy scrambled eggs	Recipe: Papaya and golden linseed smoothie	3 tbsp bran flakes and 200 ml milk	2 slices granary toast with 2 tbsp peanut butter
Mid-morning snack		Boiled egg	15 grapes and 1 handful cashews	
Lunch	Recipe: Zingy smoked salmon salad with avocado 3 celery sticks and 1 tbsp cottage cheese	Recipe: Chinese vegetable soup with tofu	Recipe: Creamy mushroom soup, served with: ham (4 medium slices) and salad Wholemeal bread roll (large) with low-fat spread (1 tsp)	Recipe: White bean salad with hard-boiled eggs, served with: 4 wholemeal crackers and 1 tbsp low-fat cream cheese
Mid-afternoon snack	30 g piece of Edam	Handful of Brazil nuts	Two satsumas	Handful of Brazil nuts
Evening meal	Recipe: Tangy chicken drumsticks with crudités and a harissa dip	Recipe: White fish with tangy watercress sauce, served with: 4 tbsp steamed vegetables Small pot of diet yoghurt	Recipe: Prawns with beans, tomatoes and thyme, served with: 4 tbsp cooked brown rice	Recipe: Marinated lamb and red onion kebabs with a yoghurt and herb sauce, served with: 1 wholemeal pitta Large salad Recipe: Apricot and apple fruit salad
Supper	Handful of pistachio nuts	7 cherry tomatoes and 10 olives	Oatcake and 1 tbsp low-fat hummus	
Drinks	200 ml milk in drinks throughout the day	200 ml milk in drinks throughout the day	200 ml milk in drinks throughout the day	200 ml milk in drinks throughout the day

Week 2 Friday–Sunday

Meal	Friday	Saturday	Sunday
Breakfast	2 wheat or oat 'bisk' cereal with 200 ml milk	1 kipper fillet with 2 slices wholemeal toast and 2 tsp low-fat spread	2 rashers grilled bacon, 1 poached egg and 1 slice of wholemeal toast with 1 tsp low-fat spread
Mid-morning snack	1 small (3 tbsp), low-fat fromage frais	Orange	Pear
Lunch	2 slices of Granary toast with 2 tsp low-fat spread and a tin of sardines in tomato sauce Glass of vegetable juice	Recipe: Horiatiki salata – Greek salad served with: 4 tbsp cooked wholemeal pasta	Recipe: Courgette soup with basil and a tomato salsa, and a chicken (3 slices) and salad (1 bowl) sandwich on a wholemeal roll with 1 tbsp low-fat mayonnaise
Mid-afternoon snack	Small apple and clementine	20 g unsweetened popcorn	Pepper sticks with 1 tbsp low-fat hummus
Evening meal	Recipe: Courgette frittata, served with baked potato (240 g) and a large salad with 1 tbsp mixed salad beans Recipe: Yoghurt ice cream with raspberries	Recipe: Healthy chicken tagine, served with 4 tbsp cooked wholemeal couscous	Recipe: Roasted vegetables with grilled halloumi (see page 90), served with homemade potato wedges (240 g) baked in olive oil
Supper	Carrot sticks and 1 tbsp low-fat hummus	One small yoghurt (150–200 g)	Handful of unsalted peanuts
Drinks	200 ml milk in drinks throughout the day	200 ml milk in drinks throughout the day	200 ml milk in drinks throughout the day

Week 1 (vegetarian) Monday–Thursday

Meal	Monday	Tuesday	Wednesday	Thursday
Breakfast	One poached egg, ½ tin plum tomatoes and 1 vegetarian sausage	Recipe: One-dish baked egg, spinach and mushroom	2 wheat or oat 'bisk' cereal with 200 ml milk and 1 tbsp dried fruit	Recipe: Porridge with dried fruit
Mid-morning snack	100 g tofu strips sautéed in spices		Handful of pistachios	1 boiled egg
Lunch	Recipe: Cauliflower soup	Vegetable sticks (½ green pepper and one stick celery) with 2 tbsp low-fat hummus and 30 g slice of low-fat cream cheese	Recipe: Courgette soup with basil and a tomato salsa with 2 oatcakes and 2 tbsp low-fat hummus	4 Rye crispbreads with 1 tbsp low-fat cream cheese plus mixed salad (one bowl green salad plus other veg)with 4½ tbsp salad beans and olive oil low-fat dressing
Mid-afternoon snack	30 g piece of low-fat cheese	Handful of mixed nuts	Apple	200 ml glass of vegetable juice
Evening meal	Recipe: Oriental vegetable stir-fry with marinated tofu and cashews 3 tbsp stewed rhubarb with sweeteners added to taste. Served with 2 tbsp natural yoghurt	Recipe: Italian bean stew 7 strawberries	Recipe: Pasta Arrabbiata with 200 g tofu, served with 2–3 tbsp steamed vegetables One small yoghurt	Recipe: Homemade classic burgers (V alternative) with 240 g homemade potato wedges, 1 tomato, salad leaves and ½ avocado Recipe: Yoghurt ice cream with raspberries
Supper	Handful of unsalted peanuts	1 boiled egg	10 olives	Handful of Brazil nuts
Drinks	200 ml milk in drinks throughout the day	200 ml milk in drinks throughout the day	200 ml milk in drinks throughout the day	200 ml milk in drinks throughout the day

Week 1 (vegetarian) Friday–Sunday

Meal	Friday	Saturday	Sunday
Breakfast	2 slices granary toast and 2 tsp olive spread with 2 grilled vegetarian sausages, one large grilled tomato and 14 button mushrooms fried in 1 dsp olive oil 200 ml glass of orange juice	Recipe: Classic muesli	2 slices wholemeal toast, 2 tsp olive spread and low-sugar jam
Mid-morning snack	30 g roast soya bean	1 plum	An apricot
Lunch	Recipe: Lentil soup with spinach and a touch of lemon, served with an oatcake or a slice of wholemeal bread and olive spread	2 slices of rye toast with 2 tsp low-fat spread and 6 tbsp baked beans	1 boiled egg and butter bean (4½ tbsp) pasta salad (4 tbsp cooked) (lettuce, spring onions and tomatoes) with 1 tsp olive oil dressing
Mid-afternoon snack	Low-fat fruit yoghurt	1 tbsp low-fat hummus with celery (one stick), cucumber (5 cm) and carrot (one whole) crudités	
Evening meal	Homemade pizza – use a small wholemeal pizza base and 1 tbsp tomato purée, olive oil and garlic base with vegetables (onions, peppers, sweetcorn, mushrooms, olives) and 30 g mozzarella cheese on top. Serve with large mixed salad	Recipe: White bean salad with hard-boiled eggs, served with 240g new potatoes and 7 cherry tomatoes Satsuma	Recipe: Aubergine curry with chickpeas, rice and a mango raita Recipe: Prune delight, served with 3 tbsp low-fat Greek yoghurt
Supper	Peach	One small yoghurt	30 g roast soya beans
Drinks	200 ml milk in drinks throughout the day	200 ml milk in drinks throughout the day	200 ml milk in drinks throughout the day

Week 2 (vegetarian) Monday–Thursday

Meal	Monday	Tuesday	Wednesday	Thursday
Breakfast	Half a grapefruit Recipe: Spicy scrambled eggs	Recipe: Papaya and golden linseed smoothie	Scrambled egg (2 eggs) and ½ a tin of plum tomatoes on 2 slices of rye toast and 2 tsp low-fat spread 200 ml glass of milk	1 poached egg and 1 vegetarian sausage with 2 slices granary toast with 1 tsp low-fat spread
Mid-morning snack	30 g piece of Edam	2 boiled eggs		
Lunch	Recipe: Mint, feta and soya bean salad	Recipe: Chinese vegetable soup with tofu	Recipe: Creamy mushroom soup, served with: 4 wholemeal crackers and 1 tbsp low-fat hummus 4 almonds	Recipe: White bean salad with hard-boiled eggs, served with: 2 oatcakes and 1 tbsp low-fat soft white cheese
Mid-afternoon snack	Handful of Brazil nuts	Vegetable sticks (one carrot) and 1 tbsp low-fat hummus	Pear	7 cherry tomatoes
Evening meal	Recipe: Ginger, soy and chilli tofu skewers with Chinese leaf and mangetout salad	Recipe: Mushroom stew with thyme and feta	Recipe: Bean and green pepper chilli, served with a green salad 7 strawberries One small yoghurt	Recipe: Crunchy stuffed peppers with rocket and raita Recipe: Apricot and apple fruit salad
Supper	One small diet yoghurt	Handful of mixed unsalted nuts	30 g roasted soya beans	200 ml glass of milk
Drinks	200 ml milk in drinks throughout the day	200 ml milk in drinks throughout the day	200 ml milk in drinks throughout the day	200 ml milk in drinks throughout the day

Week 2 (vegetarian) Friday–Sunday

Meal	Friday	Saturday	Sunday
Breakfast	2 wheat or oat 'bisk' cereal with 200 ml milk 200 ml glass of fruit juice	2 slices wholemeal toast with 1 tsp low-fat spread served with 2 poached eggs	Recipe: Porridge with dried fruit
Mid-morning snack	1 small pot low-fat fromage frais		2 plums
Lunch	Recipe: Roasted tomato soup with pesto, served with 2 oatcakes and 2 tbsp low-fat hummus and cucumber crudités	Recipe: Horiatiki salata – Greek salad, served with 1 wholemeal pitta	Recipe: Bean and green pepper chilli, served with 1 large baked potato instead of rice
Mid-afternoon snack	Banana	Apple	1 tbsp each of low-fat cream cheese and hummus with 2 large carrots
Evening meal	Bean and vegetable bake (Adapted recipe: Prawns with beans, tomatoes and thyme – make without prawns and instead soften onions and peppers in the oil before adding the tomatoes, and serve with a mashed potato topping (240 g) and a green salad	Recipe: Courgette frittata, served with 1 small baked potato and mixed salad with 2 tbsp butter beans Recipe: Brown rice pudding	Recipe: Ginger, soy and chilli tofu skewers with Chinese leaf and mangetout salad with 2 tbsp cooked brown rice
Supper	A handful of mixed nuts	1 satsuma	A handful of Brazil nuts and roast soya beans
Drinks	200 ml milk in drinks throughout the day	200 ml milk in drinks throughout the day	200 ml milk in drinks throughout the day

Appendix D: Ready Reckoners

Use these tables to look up how many calories or portions of foods you can have a day according to your gender, age and current weight. They include both information for weight loss and information for weight maintenance.

▶ Energy requirements have been determined based on your gender, age and current weight. You will lose weight quicker if you also follow an exercise plan.

▶ It is important to get adequate protein, dairy, fruit and vegetables on the two diet and five non-diet days of The 2-Day Diet. This is why there are minimum amounts for protein, and recommended amounts for dairy, fruit and vegetables each day. Having enough protein helps you to maintain your muscle mass when you are dieting.

▶ You do not need to eat the maximum amounts in the table. However, it is important to get the balance of foods right. For example if you only have two-thirds of your maximum protein portions, you should also roughly aim for two-thirds of your maximum fat and high-fibre carbohydrate portions.

Ready reckoner | Weight loss | Males
Up to 12½ stone (79 kg)

	2 diet days	5 non-diet days														
		Less than 8½ stone (54 kg)			8½–9½ stone (54–60 kg)			9½–10½ stone (60–67 kg)			10½–11½ stone (67–73 kg)			11½–12½ stone (73–79 kg)		
		Age 18–29	Age 30–60	Age 60+	Age 18–29	Age 30–60	Age 60+	Age 18–29	Age 30–60	Age 60+	Age 18–29	Age 30–60	Age 60+	Age 18–29	Age 30–60	Age 60+
Maximum kcal per day	1,100	1,600	1,600	1,400	1,700	1,600	1,400	1,900	1,800	1,600	2,000	1,900	1,700	2,100	2,000	1,800
Carbohydrate servings	0	Max 7	Min 3	Max 6	Max 7	Max 7	Max 6	Max 8	Max 8	Min 5	Max 9	Max 9	Max 7	Max 11	Max 9	Max 8
Protein servings	Min 4	Min 3	Min 3	Min 3	Min 4	Min 4	Min 4	Min 5	Min 5	Min 5	Min 6	Min 6	Min 6	Min 7	Min 7	Min 7
	Max 14	Max 9	Max 9	Max 8	Max 10	Max 9	Max 8	Max 12	Max 11	Max 9	Max 14	Max 12	Max 10	Max 14	Max 14	Max 11
Fat servings	Max 6	Max 4	Max 4	Max 3	Max 5	Max 4	Max 3	Max 5	Max 5	Max 4	Max 5	Max 5	Max 5	Max 5	Max 5	Max 5
Dairy servings	3 (recommended)	3 (recommended for all weight groups)														
Vegetable servings	5 (recommended)	5 (recommended for all weight groups)														
Fruit servings	1 (recommended)	2 (recommended for all weight groups)														

Ready reckoner | Weight loss | Males

Over 12½ stone (79 kg)

	2 diet days	5 non-diet days											
		12½–13½ stone (79–86 kg)			13½–14½ stone (86–92 kg)			14½–15½ stone (92–98 kg)			Above 15½ stone (98 kg)		
		Age 18–29	Age 30–60	Age 60+	Age 18–29	Age 30–60	Age 60+	Age 18–29	Age 30–60	Age 60+	Age 18–29	Age 30–60	Age 60+
Maximum kcal per day	1,100	2,300	2,200	2,000	2,500	2,300	2,100	2,500	2,400	2,200	2,500	2,500	2,300
Carbohydrate servings	0	Max 12	Max 11	Max 9	Max 13	Max 12	Max 11	Max 13	Max 12	Max 11	Max 13	Max 13	Max 12
Protein servings	Min 4	Min 8	Min 8	Min 8	Min 9	Min 9	Min 9	Min 10	Min 10	Min 10	Min 11	Min 11	Min 11
	Max 14	Max 16	Max 15	Max 14	Max 17	Max 16	Max 14	Max 17	Max 17	Max 15	Max 17	Max 17	Max 16
Fat servings	Max 6	Max 6	Max 5	Max 5	Max 7	Max 6	Max 5	Max 7	Max 6	Max 5	Max 7	Max 7	Max 6
Dairy servings	3 (recommended)	3 (recommended for all weight groups)											
Vegetable servings	5 (recommended)	5 (recommended for all weight groups)											
Fruit servings	1 (recommended)	2 (recommended for all weight groups)											

Ready reckoner | Weight loss | Females
Up to 12½ stone (79 kg)

	2 diet days	5 non-diet days														
		Less than 8½ stone (54 kg)			8½–9½ stone (54–60 kg)			9½–10½ stone (60–67 kg)			10½–11½ stone (67–73 kg)			11½–12½ stone (73–79 kg)		
		Age 18–29	Age 30–60	Age 60+	Age 18–29	Age 30–60	Age 60+	Age 18–29	Age 30–60	Age 60+	Age 18–29	Age 30–60	Age 60+	Age 18–29	Age 30–60	Age 60+
Maximum kcal per day	1,000	1,500	1,400	1,400	1,500	1,400	1,400	1,700	1,500	1,400	1,800	1,600	1,500	1,900	1,700	1,600
Carbohydrate servings	0	Max 6	Max 6	Max 6	Max 6	Max 6	Max 6	Max 7	Max 6	Max 6	Max 8	Max 7	Max 6	Max 9	Max 7	Max 7
Protein servings	Min 4	Min 3	Min 3	Min 3	Min 4	Min 4	Min 4	Min 5	Min 5	Min 5	Min 6	Min 6	Min 6	Min 7	Min 7	Min 7
	Max 12	Max 8	Max 8	Max 8	Max 8	Max 8	Max 8	Max 10	Max 8	Max 8	Max 11	Max 9	Max 8	Max 12	Max 10	Max 9
Fat servings	Max 5	Max 4	Max 3	Max 3	Max 4	Max 3	Max 3	Max 5	Max 4	Max 3	Max 5	Max 4	Max 4	Max 5	Max 5	Max 4
Dairy servings	3 (recommended)	3 (recommended for all weight groups)														
Vegetable servings	5 (recommended)	5 (recommended for all weight groups)														
Fruit servings	1 (recommended)	2 (recommended for all weight groups)														

Ready reckoner | Weight loss | Females
Over 12½ stone (79 kg)

	2 diet days	5 non-diet days												
		12½–13½ stone (79–86 kg)			13½–14½ stone (86–92 kg)			14½–15½ stone (92–98 kg)			Above 15½ stone (98 kg)		
		Age 18–29	Age 30–60	Age 60+	Age 18–29	Age 30–60	Age 60+	Age 18–29	Age 30–60	Age 60+	Age 18–29	Age 30–60	Age 60+
Maximum kcal per day	1,000	2,000	1,800	1,700	2,000	1,900	1,800	2,000	2,000	1,800	2,000	2,000	1,900
Carbohydrate servings	0	Max 9	Max 8	Max 7	Max 9	Max 9	Max 8	Max 9	Max 9	Max 8	Max 9	Max 9	Max 9
Protein servings	Min 4	Min 8	Min 8	Min 8	Min 9	Min 9	Min 9	Min 10	Min 10	Min 9	Min 11	Min 11	Min 11
	Max 12	Max 14	Max 11	Max 10	Max 14	Max 12	Max 11	Max 14	Max 14	Max 11	Max 14	Max 14	Max 12
Fat servings	Max 5	Max 5	Max 5	Max 5	Max 5	Max 5	Max 5	Max 5	Max 5	Max 5	Max 5	Max 5	Max 5
Dairy servings	3 (recommended)	3 (recommended for all weight groups)											
Vegetable servings	5 (recommended)	5 (recommended for all weight groups)											
Fruit servings	1 (recommended)	2 (recommended for all weight groups)											

Ready reckoner | Weight maintenance | Males
Up to 11½ stone (73 kg)

	1 diet day	Less than 8½ stone (54 kg)			8½–9½ stone (54–60 kg)			9½–10½ stone (60–67 kg)			10½–11½ stone (67–73 kg)		
		Age 18–29	Age 30–60	Age 60+	Age 18–29	Age 30–60	Age 60+	Age 18–29	Age 30–60	Age 60+	Age 18–29	Age 30–60	Age 60+
Maximum kcal per day	1,100	1,900	1,800	1,600	2,000	1,900	1,700	2,100	2,000	1,800	2,300	2,200	2,000
Carbohydrate servings	0	Max 8	Max 8	Max 7	Max 9	Max 9	Max 7	Max 11	Max 9	Max 8	Max 12	Max 11	Max 9
Protein servings	Min 4	Min 3	Min 3	Min 3	Min 4	Min 4	Min 4	Min 5	Min 5	Min 5	Min 6	Min 6	Min 6
	Max 14	Max 12	Max 11	Max 9	Max 14	Max 12	Max 10	Max 14	Max 14	Max 11	Max 16	Max 15	Max 14
Fat servings	Max 6	Max 5	Max 5	Max 4	Max 5	Max 5	Max 5	Max 5	Max 5	Max 5	Max 6	Max 5	Max 5
Dairy servings	3 (recommended)	3 (recommended for all weight groups)											
Vegetable servings	5 (recommended)	5 (recommended for all weight groups)											
Fruit servings	1 (recommended)	2 (recommended for all weight groups)											

Ready reckoner | Weight maintenance | Males
Over 11½ stone (73 kg)

	1 diet day	6 non-diet days											
		11½–12½ stone (73–79 kg)			12½–13½ stone (79–86 kg)			13½–14½ stone (86–92 kg)			Above 14½ stone (92 kg)		
		Age 18–29	Age 30–60	Age 60+	Age 18–29	Age 30–60	Age 60+	Age 18–29	Age 30–60	Age 60+	Age 18–29	Age 30–60	Age 60+
Maximum kcal per day	1,100	2,400	2,300	2,100	2,500	2,400	2,200	2,500	2,500	2,300	2,500	2,500	2,500
Carbohydrate servings	0	Max 12	Max 12	Max 11	Max 13	Max 12	Max 11	Max 13	Max 13	Max 12	Max 13	Max 13	Max 13
Protein servings	Min 4	Min 7	Min 7	Min 7	Min 8	Min 8	Min 8	Min 9	Min 9	Min 9	Min 10	Min 10	Min 10
	Max 14	Max 17	Max 16	Max 14	Max 17	Max 17	Max 15	Max 17	Max 17	Max 16	Max 17	Max 17	Max 17
Fat servings	Max 6	Max 6	Max 6	Max 5	Max 7	Max 6	Max 5	Max 7	Max 7	Max 6	Max 7	Max 7	Max 7
Dairy servings	3 (recommended)	3 (recommended for all weight groups)											
Vegetable servings	5 (recommended)	5 (recommended for all weight groups)											
Fruit servings	1 (recommended)	2 (recommended for all weight groups)											

Ready reckoner | Weight maintenance | Females
Up to 11½ stone (73 kg)

	1 diet day	6 non-diet days											
		Less than 8½ stone (54 kg)			8½–9½ stone (54–60 kg)			9½–10½ stone (60–67 kg)			10½–11½ stone (67–73 kg)		
		Age 18–29	Age 30–60	Age 60+	Age 18–29	Age 30–60	Age 60+	Age 18–29	Age 30–60	Age 60+	Age 18–29	Age 30–60	Age 60+
Maximum kcal per day	1,000	1,700	1,600	1,500	1,800	1,700	1,500	1,900	1,800	1,600	2,000	1,900	1,700
Carbohydrate servings	0	Max 7	Max 7	Max 6	Max 8	Max 7	Max 6	Max 9	Max 8	Max 7	Max 9	Max 9	Max 7
Protein servings	Min 4	Min 3	Min 3	Min 3	Min 4	Min 4	Min 4	Min 5	Min 5	Min 5	Min 6	Min 6	Min 6
	Max 12	Max 10	Max 9	Max 8	Max 11	Max 10	Max 8	Max 12	Max 11	Max 9	Max 14	Max 12	Max 10
Fat servings	Max 5	Max 5	Max 4	Max 4	Max 5	Max 5	Max 4	Max 5	Max 5	Max 4	Max 5	Max 5	Max 5
Dairy servings	3 (recommended)	3 (recommended for all weight groups)											
Vegetable servings	5 (recommended)	5 (recommended for all weight groups)											
Fruit servings	1 (recommended)	2 (recommended for all weight groups)											

Ready reckoner | Weight maintenance | Females
Over 11½ stone (73 kg)

	1 diet day	6 non-diet days											
		11½–12½ stone (73–79 kg)			12½–13½ stone (79–86 kg)			13½–14½ stone (86–92 kg)			Above 14½ stone (92 kg)		
		Age 18–29	Age 30–60	Age 60+	Age 18–29	Age 30–60	Age 60+	Age 18–29	Age 30–60	Age 60+	Age 18–29	Age 30–60	Age 60+
Maximum kcal per day	1,000	2,000	1,900	1,800	2,000	2,000	1,900	2,000	2,000	2,000	2,000	2,000	2,000
Carbohydrate servings	0	Max 9	Max 9	Max 8	Max 9	Max 9	Max 9	Max 9	Max 9	Max 9	Max 9	Max 9	Max 9
Protein servings	Min 4 / Max 12	Min 7 / Max 14	Min 7 / Max 12	Min 7 / Max 11	Min 8 / Max 14	Min 8 / Max 14	Min 8 / Max 12	Min 9 / Max 14	Min 9 / Max 14	Min 9 / Max 14	Min 10 / Max 14	Min 10 / Max 14	Min 10 / Max 14
Fat servings	Max 5	Max 5	Max 5	Max 5	Max 5	Max 5	Max 5	Max 5	Max 5	Max 5	Max 5	Max 5	Max 5
Dairy servings	3 (recommended)	3 (recommended for all weight groups)											
Vegetable servings	5 (recommended)	5 (recommended for all weight groups)											
Fruit servings	1 (recommended)	2 (recommended for all weight groups)											

References

Chapter 1 references

1   http://www.ons.gov.uk/ons/relldisability-and-health-measurement/
    health-expectancies-at-birth-and-age-65-in-the-united-kingdom/
    2008–10/stb-he-2008-2010.html

2   Harvie MN, Howell A et al., 'Association of gain and loss of weight
    before and after menopause with risk of postmenopausal breast cancer
    in the Iowa women's health study', *Cancer Epidemiology, Biomarkers &
    Prevention*, 14/3 (2005), 656–661.

3   Wing RR et al., 'Long-term weight loss maintenance', *The American
    Journal of Clinical Nutrition*, 82/1 Suppl (2005), 222S–225S.

4   Cleary MP et al., 'Weight-cycling decreases incidence and increases
    latency of mammary tumors to a greater extent than does chronic caloric
    restriction in mouse mammary tumor virus-transforming growth factor-
    alpha female mice', *Cancer Epidemiology, Biomarkers & Prevention*,
    11/9, (2002), 836–43.

5   Anson RM, Mattson MP et al., 'Intermittent fasting dissociates beneficial
    effects of dietary restriction on glucose metabolism and neuronal resis-
    tance to injury from calorie intake', Proceedings of the National Academy
    of Sciences of the United States of America, 100/10 (2003), 6216–20.

6   Harvie M, et al. The effect of intermittent energy and carbohydrate
    restriction v. daily energy restriction on weight loss and metabolic
    disease risk markers in overweight women. *Br J Nutr* 2013;1–14.

7   Willett WC, 'The Mediterranean Diet: Science and practice', Public
    Health Nutr, 9/1A (2006), 105–10.

8   Redman LM, et al. (2009). Metabolic and behavioral compensations
    in response to caloric restriction: implications for the maintenance of
    weight loss. *PLoS One* 4: e4377.

9   Garrow JS, Summerbell CD (1995) Meta-analysis: effect of exercise,
    with or without dieting, on the body composition of overweight
    subjects. *Eur J Clin Nutr* 49: 1–10.

10 Gill JM, Hardman AE, Exercise and postprandial lipid metabolism: an
    update on potential mechanisms and interactions with high-carbohy-
    drate diets, *J Nutr Biochem* (2003), Mar; 14(3): 122–32.

11 Byberg L, et al. (2009) Total mortality after changes in leisure time
    physical activity in 50 year old men: 35 year follow-up of population
    based cohort. *BMJ* 338: b688.

12 Lemanne D, et al., The role of physical activity in cancer prevention, treatment, recovery, and survivorship. *Oncology* (Williston Park). 2013 Jun; 27(6): 580–5.

13 Johnson F et al., 'Dietary restraint and self-regulation in eating behavior', *International Journal of Obesity* (London), 36/5 (2012), 665–674,

14 Paulweber B et al., 'A European evidence-based guideline for the prevention of type 2 diabetes', *Hormone and Metabolic Research*, 42 Suppl 1 (2010), S3–36.

15 McCullough ML, et al. Following cancer prevention guidelines reduces risk of cancer, cardiovascular disease, and all-cause mortality. Cancer Epidemiol Biomarkers Prev. 2011 Jun; 20(6):1089–97. doi: 10.1158/1055–9965.EPI-10-1173. Epub 2011 Apr 5. PubMed PMID: 21467238.

16 Hirsch, AR et al., 'Effect of Television Viewing on Sensory-Specific Satiety: Are Leno and Letterman Obesogenic?', 89th Annual Meeting Endocrine Society (Abstract) (2007).

17 Baldwin KM et al., 'Effects of weight loss and leptin on skeletal muscle in human subjects', *The American Journal of Physiology – Regulatory, Integrative and Comparative Physiology*, 301/5 (2011), R1259–R1266.

Chapter 2 references

1 Carlson O, et al. Impact of reduced meal frequency without caloric restriction on glucose regulation in healthy, normal-weight middle-aged men and women. *Metabolism* 2007; 56(12):1729–1734.

2 Smeets AJ et al., 'Acute effects on metabolism and appetite profile of one meal difference in the lower range of meal frequency', *British Journal of Nutrition*, 99/6 (2008), 1316–1321.

3 Holmback U et al., 'The human body may buffer small differences in meal size and timing during a 24-hour wake period provided energy balance is maintained', *British Journal of Nutrition*, 133/9 (2003), 2748–55.

4 Halsey LG et al., 'Does consuming breakfast influence activity levels? An experiment into the effect of breakfast consumption on eating habits and energy expenditure', *Public Health Nutrition*, 15/2 (2012), 238–245.

5 Brinkworth GD et al., 'Effects of a low carbohydrate weight loss diet on exercise capacity and tolerance in obese subjects'. *Obesity* (Silver Spring), 17/10 (2009), 1916–1923.

6 Estruch R, et al. PREDIMED Study Investigators. Primary prevention of cardiovascular disease with a Mediterranean diet. N Engl J Med. 2013 Apr 4;368(14): 1279–90.

References

7   Chobanian AV, et al. Seventh report of the Joint National Committee on Prevention, Detection, Evaluation, and Treatment of High Blood Pressure. *Hypertension* 2003; 42(6):1206–1252.

8   Lieberman HR, et al. A double-blind, placebo-controlled test of two days calorie deprivation: effects on cognition, activity, sleep, and interstitial glucose concentrations. *Am J Clin Nutr* 2008; 88(3):667–676.

9   Brinkworth GD, et al. Long-term effects of a very low-carbohydrate diet and a low-fat diet on mood and cognitive function. *Arch Intern Med* 2009; 169(20):1873–1880. {D'Anci, Watts, et al. 2009 181 /id}

10 Krikorian R, et al. Dietary ketosis enhances memory in mild cognitive impairment. *Neurobiol Aging* 2012; 33(2):425–427.

11 King NA et al., 'Individual variability following 12 weeks of supervised exercise: identification and characterization of compensation for exercise-induced weight loss'. *International Journal of Obesity*, 32 (2008), 177–184.

12 Mason C et al., 'History of weight cycling does not impede future weight loss or metabolic improvements in postmenopausal women', *Metabolism*, 62/1 (2013), 127–36.

13 Hall KD et al., 'Quantification of the effect of energy imbalance on bodyweight', *The Lancet*, 378/9793 (2011), 826–837.

14 May et al., 'Elaborated Intrusion Theory: A Cognitive-Emotional Theory of Food Craving', Current Obesity Reports, 1 (2012), 114–121.

15 Campagne DM, 'The premenstrual syndrome revisited', *European Journal of Obstetrics & Gynecology and Reproductive Biology*, 130/1 (2007), 4–17.

16 Wing RR et al., 'Prescribed "breaks" as a means to disrupt weight control efforts', *Obesity Research*, 11/2 (2003), 287–291.

Acknowledgements

Many thanks to Anne Montague, Jo Godfrey Wood and Mary Pegington, for editing the manuscript; Kate Santon and Emily Jonzen for devising the recipes; Kath Sellers for analysing and collating the recipes for the book and Grace Cooper for helping devise the meal plans. Thanks also to Alan Rosenthal and Mark Seymour-Mead at steweduk.co.uk for adapting one of their delicious stew recipes for diet days. Our thanks also to Debbie McMullan and Rebecca Dodd-Chandler for their advice and expertise and the illustrator, Stephen Dew for the exercise advice and illustrations, which can be found at www.thetwodaydiet.co.uk.

This book has evolved from our intermittent diet research. We thank our collaborators and colleagues who have made this work possible. Firstly Mark Mattson from the National Institute on Ageing, Baltimore, and Margot Cleary from The University of Minnesota for sharing insights from their research, which inspired us to undertake our dietary studies. Secondly the team of scientists and researchers who have helped run these studies: Gareth Evans, Claire Wright, Ellen Mitchell, Lesley Coates, Helen Sumner, Rosemary Greenhalgh, Jenny Affen, Jayne Beesley at The Nightingale Centre and Genesis Breast Cancer Prevention.

We are grateful to the rest of Mark Mattson's team including Bronwen Martin and Roy Cutler, Jan Frystyk and Alan Flyvbjerg (Arhus University Hospital, Denmark), Roy Goodacre, Andrew Vaughan, Will Allwood, Robert Clarke, Kath Spence (all University of Manchester), Andy Sims

(University of Edinburgh), Wendy Russell (Rowett Institute) who have all helped to assess the impact of the diets on the body and disease risk. Thanks also to the following individuals for their invaluable advice: Susan Jebb (weight management), Julie Morris (statistics) and Louise Donnelly (health psychology and dieting behaviours).

Our greatest thanks are to Lester Barr, Pam Glass, Geoff Swarbrick, the Genesis Breast Cancer Prevention trustees who have consistently supported our dietary research for the past 11 years. Also Nikki Hoffman, Michelle Cohen, the Genesis office team and the Genesis volunteers who give up their time to help us in the office and run research clinics, particularly Jane Eaton, Susan Roe, Pauline Sadler, Philippa Quirk, Louise Blacklock, Alison Rees and Angela Foster. Thanks also to Amy Tao and Matthew Collier, our Genesis graduate interns.

We thank the numerous dieters who have worked with us on the studies over the past 12 years, without whom none of the research would be possible. Also staff within The Nightingale Centre and Genesis Breast Cancer Prevention and University Hospital South Manchester who have been successfully dieting with our 2-Day Diet and inspired us to write this book.

Finally Susanna Abbott and Catherine Knight at Ebury for their patience and hard work in making this book.

Recipe credits

All recipes by Kate Santon except for the following:

Emily Jonzen on pages 76, 91–2, 102, 115–16, 120–1, 134

Stewed! on page 93.

Index

Index

Index

Index

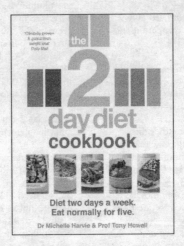
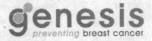